TRAINING YOURSELF
A Complete Encyclopedia for Getting Your Body & Mind Into Great Shape

Kris Gebhardt

GCI Press

Published by GCI Press
Indianapolis, IN

© 2000 Kris Gebhardt
All rights reserved. Published 2000

Printed in the United States of America.

No part of this publication may be reproduced, stored in a retrieval system, or transmitted, in any form or by any means, electronic, mechanical, photocopying, recording, or otherwise, without the prior permission of Kris Gebhardt.

99 00 01 02 03 04   10 9 8 7 6 5 4 3 2 1

Library of Congress Cataloging-in-Publication Data pending

The author and publisher assume no responsibility for any injury that may occur as a result of attempting to do any of the movements, techniques or exercises described in this book. This book requires strenuous physical activity and a physical examination is advisable before starting this or any other exercise program.

for mom

---

to JCM

thanks for the advice:

*Suck it up and
tough it out and
do the best you can.*

Credits

Cover designer—Phil Velikan

Cover photographer—Garry Chilluffo

Photographer—Karen Huckabone

Photographer—Chuck Gebhardt

Editor and book designer—Heather Lowhorn

Proofreader—Deborah Lilly

Equipment Supplier—Pete Grimmer and Chris Lynch, Pro Industries

Special thanks...

to Elaine Mellencamp for modeling the exercises.

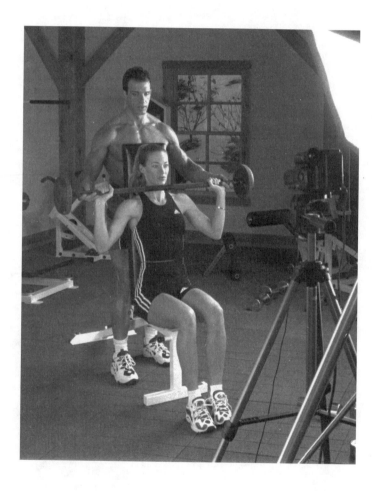

Foreword

Phyllis McCullough
President and CEO, Cook Inc.

It all started simply enough. It was December, 1997, and I was hosting a dinner party. John and Elaine Mellencamp were there, and John was showing off his physique. I'll admit he was in great shape-better than I had ever seen him. After a scare with some heart problems, John had really started to take care of his body. Still, I couldn't resist ribbing him.

"Sure," I said, "Anybody could get in great shape with their own workout room and personal trainer." John isn't one to back down from a challenge, so after a little good-natured teasing back and forth, he cut to the chase. He bet me that I wouldn't stick with a workout program for a full year, even with the use of his workout room and his personal trainer. I told him he was on.

That's how I met Kris Gebhardt. He had been the Mellencamp's trainer for some time, and because of the bet, he was about to become mine. By January I was sitting in the Mellencamp's training room with Kris. It was the beginning of a whole new outlook on wellness and physical fitness for me. I realized having equipment and a trainer wasn't going to magically get me in shape. I still had a lot of effort to contribute, but I was not going to lose that bet.

I help run one of the world's largest manufacturers and distributors of medical products. As you can guess, I am busy. I don't have a lot of time to spend in a gym. Kris understood that, and he developed a program that fit into my life. We began meeting two to three times a week on my lunch hours. I found myself really enjoying it. It felt great to get out of the office. I ate less at lunch, plus I could feel the difference in my body.

To make a long story short, I won that bet. In fact, somewhere along the way, it stopped being about the bet. Has my life improved since I started working with Kris? Definitely. I am still working out two years later because of the improvements Kris' insights into training have brought into my life. My self-esteem is better; I have more stamina; I deal with stress more efficiently.

And I'm not the only one Kris has helped at Cook Inc. My boss, Bill Cook, owner of the company, began experiencing heart trouble in early 1999. John and I knew Kris could turn Bill's health around. We ganged up on him and told him how working with Kris would change his life. Of course, we were right. Like John's, Bill's heart troubles—and his general health—are vastly improved.

When the Mellencamps moved to a new house farther from our office, Bill and I had exercise equipment installed at the office so we could continue to workout at lunch. It wasn't long before others at the company began to join us in our workouts. That led to a great idea: Why not build an exercise facility that would be available to all our employees? But not just a room with some weights. We knew that, like ourselves, our employees would only really benefit from such a facility if they new how to set goals for themselves, develop proper training programs to meet those goals, and motivate themselves. In short, all the things Kris had taught us. We didn't want our employees to be left on their own to stumble around with the weights for a couple of months only to become frustrated and then quit. We turned to Kris for help.

And help me did. He designed a fabulous, state-of-the-art facility. We plan to open the facility in a couple of weeks, and Kris will be involved in training the gym staff to help our employees. We believe happier, healthier employees are great for business. That is why we felt this was so important. That is why we have invested in this facility. And that is why we are relying on Kris.

Kris is not about the short term or immediate results. He is about the whole picture. He is a tremendous talent in his field because he has a passion for educating people about training. Fortunately, he has written books such as this one so we can all learn his methods. Whether you are a pregnant woman, an older man with health problems, or a healthy person who wants to look better, Kris can show you how to develop your body into exactly what you want. And not just for today, but for a lifetime.

Thanks, Kris. That was the best bet I ever made.

Contents

Introduction 1

Part One
Training For Health, Fitness, and More 5
Training Yourself 7
Setting Up A Successful Training Program 15
Training Anatomy 23
Aerobic Training 29
The Basics Of Weight Training 35
The Basics Of Nutrition 39
The Importance Of Supplements 47
Secrets Of Training Longevity 51
Stretching And Flexibility 53
Beginning Weight Training Program 59
Intermediate Weight Training 71
Advanced Level Weight Training 87
Training For Safe Weight Loss 113
Training For Fat-Free Weight Gain 135
Injury and Overtraining 149
Training And Pregnancy 153
Training After Pregnancy 167
Figure Firming For Women 179
Shaping Up Without Weights 197
The "I Just Don't Feel Like Training Today" Solution 203
Training "Under The Weather" 205

Part Two
More Great Exercises For Shaping Up 207
More Great Exercises For The Chest 209
More Great Exercises For The Back 213
More Great Exercises For The Shoulders 217
More Great Exercises For The Biceps 223
More Great Exercises For The Triceps 227
More Great Exercises For The Forearms 231
More Great Exercises For The Calves 233
More Great Exercises For The Quadriceps 235
More Great Exercises For Hips And Thighs 237
More Great Exercises For The Abdomen 239

Part Three
Training For Your Favorite Sport 243
Training For Running 245
Training For Golf 259
Training For Tennis 269

Part Four
Getting Your Mind Into Your Training 279
Develop A Training Ethic 281
Think Big... 285
Take Responsibility 287
Adjust Your Attitude 289
Goal Setting 291
Getting The Most Out Of Each Training Session 293
Supercharging Your Motivation 295

About the Author 299

Introduction

January 1985. Ann Arbor, Michigan.
5:30 a.m. It's my first day on the job working for Tom Monaghan, president and CEO of the Domino's Pizza empire. It's pitch black; a foot of snow already covers the ground and more falls silently. The temperature is 5 below; the wind chill is -20. The porch light comes on and out walks Tom in his running suit, knit hat, and gloves. I remember being so cold I could hardly get my mouth to move to say the words good morning.

Seemingly unaffected, Tom says, "Good morning. Let's run." Sixty minutes later and six miles down the road, we reach the Domino's Pizza World Headquarters. After a quick shower and change, we board the corporate helicopter and are whisked away to the airport where the Domino's private jet is waiting to rush us to Los Angeles for a full day of meetings.

The day reluctantly comes to its close around 1:00 a.m. local time—4:00 a.m. back home in Ann Arbor. A little longer and I would have been up 24 hours straight. After a few hours of sleep, I meet Tom in the hallway of the hotel. It is 6:00 a.m.

"Good morning," he says. "Let's go lift some weights." After 45 minutes of weights and six miles of jogging, we are off on another full day of meetings. An evening flight out of L.A. puts us back in Ann Arbor early the next morning. It's snowing hard, but what else is new in Michigan?

"Good night, Tom," I say. He smiles, and says, "See you in a couple hours for our run!"

March 1992. Palm Springs, California.

It's a beautiful morning; the sun is shining; the mountains are glowing in the early light. I'm standing in the gym at the Carey Grant estate—home of Frank and Christine Zane—reviewing Zane's amazing 22-year competitive career. He's won all the major bodybuilding titles—Mr. America, Mr. World, three-time Mr. Universe, and three-time Mr. Olympia.

The gym is a shrine. Magazine covers, pictures, and posters cover the walls. Trophies, medals, and medallions add to the ambiance. I'm thinking to myself, "This man is truly a living legend." Frank enters the gym. "Good morning, Kris. Ready to workout?"

Two hours later I leave the gym having completed the same workout Frank used prior to defeating Arnold Schwarzenegger in the 1968 Mr. Universe contest. I think to myself, someone forgot to tell Frank that he is 50 years old, that he has already won all the titles there are in bodybuilding, and that Arnold isn't coming out of retirement any time soon.

May 1997. On the road.

I'm on tour with singer/songwriter John Mellencamp. This week is packed with shows—two nights in Atlanta, then it's onto one-nighters in Holmdel, New Jersey; Columbia, Missouri; Philadelphia; and Pittsburgh. Next we do two shows in Boston before heading to New York.

It's late in the week. We've been getting to bed around 3:00 a.m., and we're all pretty beat. I'm usually in the hotel gym by 8:00 a.m. for my own training. By 10:30 John usually arrives with his wife, super model Elaine Irwin Mellencamp, and security director Tracy Cowles. Today he says, "Let's lift some weights." His voice is husky. He's tired and has a sore throat. Elaine's been up all night battling the flu and their two boys' pillow fights. John lies down on the bench and grabs the bar like he's training for the Olympics. Elaine steps on the treadmill and begins relentlessly pursuing the four-mile marker. Forty-five minutes into the workout, they switch. John gets the treadmill and Elaine picks up the dumbbells. Later that afternoon, we're on the plane headed for the next venue. At 8:00 p.m, John and I are back in the gym to stretch and warm up. At 9:25 p.m. it's show time!

March 1998. Southern Indiana.

It's a cool March morning, and I'm riding my bike and talking with my dad. He's walking his usual five-mile course. He turns 62 today. He's still working 12-hour days, often six days a week. He has turned down retirement a number of times. The company has tried to hire several young executives to take over some of the work load, but they keep burning out and quitting.

This month he celebrates his 43rd year with the company. In this day and age it's hard to imagine working that many years at the same place! That's dedicated service! I ask, "Dad, when are you going to retire?" He says, "Not sure. Still got the energy and drive to keep going!"

You might be thinking what I once thought: With millions of dollars in the bank and having reached the top of their fields, why aren't these people taking it easy? Why aren't they cashing it in and heading to the beach?

What do these super stars, legends, and high achievers know that the rest of us don't? I mean, come on . . .

Tom Monaghan has more money in the bank than many small countries. Why is he jogging six miles a day in sub-zero weather? John Mellencamp is already a living legend. Why is he in the gym two hours before he is scheduled to go on stage? Elaine Erwin Mellencamp has already achieved super-model stardom. Why is she still training like she is trying to make the track team? Why is Frank Zane still training with the same intensity, mental focus and determination that he had when he was preparing to face Arnold Schwarzenegger? He already beat him! And why is 62-year-old George Gebhardt getting up everyday at the crack of dawn to speed walk his 5-mile course? Isn't he supposed to be cutting back, easing his way into retirement?

Why do these people make the sacrifices? Why do they possess such dedication? And why have they made such a tremendous commitment to their training?

On the surface, the answer is obvious: They care about their health; they want to be fit.

But what's not clearly visible is that training is the secret weapon of their successes.

I know what you must be thinking. These stories can be rather humbling. These people aren't like me. They're super-achievers, superstars, the best of the best, champions. I don't have what they've got—they have that "magic" stuff.

That is exactly how I felt over a decade ago as I stood in front of the bathroom mirror of my one-room apartment, staring at a 250-pound washed-up jock.

But then I asked, "Why not me?"

What you are about to read are the secrets that I discovered and used to drastically change my body, taking it from the depths of poor health to the pinnacle of physical excellence. These are the secrets gained from 20-plus years of training experience—the secrets that I have shared with my clients that have enabled them to develop their bodies, become healthy, and reach their goals.

And what's really special about this book is that it will teach you how to use your training to enhance your life in many ways: your career, conquering life's challenges, setting and pursuing big goals, and reaching those personal milestones.

It's amazing! Look at how these superstars have developed their training programs to not only get in shape but to enhance their lives . . .

Look . . .

. . . how Tom Monaghan has used training to give himself the energy, strength, stamina, and drive to turn a $500-dollar pizza store into a billion-dollar pizza empire!

... how John Mellencamp has used training to put himself back on stage after suffering a career-threatening heart attack. He is using training to extend his legendary music career!

... how Elaine Irwin Mellencamp has used training to put herself back in front of the camera and on the covers of the Victoria's Secret catalog and *Shape* magazine—after going through two pregnancies in just two years!

... how Frank Zane, at age 52, has used training to defy Father Time, breaking new ground in the field of bodybuilding, health and fitness, and setting the standard higher and higher for physical excellence.

... how George Gebhardt has used training to become a company legend entering his sixth decade serving the same company, doing a job that would take two or even three people to perform it today's corporate world.

Obviously, these people could cash it in, sit back, and live off their past accomplishments, yet they continue pursuing goals and achieving personal milestones. They place a priority on their health and fitness. They put forth the effort, invest quality time in training each day, and taking care of their bodies. Why?

Because training gives them the winning edge!

Training Yourself contains everything you need to know to develop a training program that will enhance your entire being! You are about to learn a lot more than how to work out. You will learn how to shape-up your body and use training to give you the winning edge in life!

The really good news is you are like these super achievers. You have the potential to reach your own levels of excellence. You, too, have that "magic" stuff!

With *Training Yourself* you will be able train yourself to become a superstar!

Kris Gebhardt

Part One

Training For Health, Fitness, and More

Chapter 1
Training Yourself

Imagine for a moment how your life would change if you knew the key to health and fitness. How would you look? What would it do for your confidence, your attitude? How about your relationships, your job, your career? It's really not such a strange concept when you think about it, training beyond the physical to increase your income, excel in your career, achieve your personal goals. After all, we don't even think twice when we hear an athlete say, "I'm in training." It's common sense that winning the game, tournament, or championship requires an athlete to be in great shape. We all know athletics require physical endurance, skill, and strength. But doesn't starting a business, raising kids, writing a book, producing gold records, or building a billion-dollar empire?

Aren't our everyday lives filled with fierce competitions, championship games, and tough tournaments?

My greatest wish is that you will use *Training Yourself—A Complete Encyclopedia for Getting Your Body and Mind Into Shape* to not only master your body, fitness, and health goals, but that you will learn to use your training the way Tom Monaghan has used it to help him achieve his unbelievable financial goals, or the way John Mellencamp has used it to extend his legendary music career, or the way Elaine Irwin Mellencamp has used it to keep herself at the top of the beauty and fashion world. I have trained this executive, musician, and model. Now let me teach you what I taught them. My goal for you is that you will learn how to implement training so that you, too, will gain the edge and become a high achiever in all areas in your life.

Change Is Possible

Over 15 years ago, I stood in my bathroom staring in the mirror at the image of my overweight body. I can remember asking myself, "Why me? Why do I have to be 50 pounds overweight? Why do some people have healthy, shapely bodies while I have to wear XXL's?" I wondered if there were fundamental secrets to being healthy, fit, and in shape. Was there something that in-shape people knew that made them that way? Or was it simple fate, the luck of the gene pool draw?

You've probably had the same feelings, perhaps when you, too, were standing naked in front of your bathroom mirror. Well, such keys to health and fitness do exist. We know this because there are people who have achieved physical excellence.

As I stood in that bathroom, it dawned on me that if others could look good, feel positively about themselves, and have endless energy, then it was possible for me, too.

Remember this key point. It was possible for me, and it's possible for you.

Why I Wrote This Book

In March of 1998, I published my third book, *Training The Teenager For the Game of Their Life: The Complete Encyclopedia of Training Programs for General Fitness, Sports and Life*.

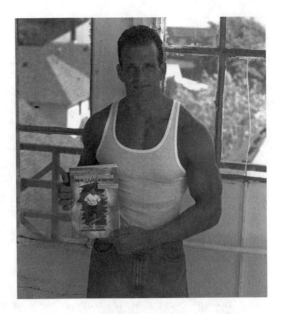

In promoting the book, I had agreed to do a book signing at Book Expo America. This trade show held annually in Chicago is the most important publishing show in the United States. It draws tens of thousands of people from all over the world. It's a five day bonanza with seminars, clinics, exhibits, meetings, and social functions.

Industry wide, publishers roll out the red carpet for the world's most famous authors who come to speak and sign autographs. These autograph sessions are a big hit and draw lots of people—if you are a big-name author. For us unknowns it usually is a humbling experience.

Although I had agreed to do the signing, I was less than eager. I was convinced it would be a waste of time. I thought, "Who is going to come into my distributor's booth to get a book by Kris Gebhardt with all those other big names nearby?"

To make matters worse, when we arrived we found ourselves sharing a booth with two players from the Chicago Bears who were promoting a book about their team. I said to my wife, "Now we are really going to get overshadowed. We are in Chicago, and those guys are local heroes. Everybody is going to go to their table. You better get set for two long, boring hours."

What happened in the next 30 minutes completely shocked me. I signed books for a nonstop line of people. I was forced to stop signing because I ran out of books! Most of the adults who stopped by my table picked up a copy for their son or daughter. But after they browsed through the book, they all asked the same question, "Can I use this myself?" They liked features such as the inclusive programs, the many photographs, the concise chapters, and the easy-to-access set up of the book.

After the book had been out for several months, I found that parents who were initially buying the book for the important teenagers in their lives were commandeering it for their own use. The comments kept coming back to me: "How about the adults? Why don't you write a book like this for adults?"

So I did!

The Role A Book Can Play

With only so many hours in a day, it's impossible for me to work individually with everyone that I get requests from. Likewise, there are many people who don't have the resources or the flexibility in their schedule to participate in one-on-one training sessions. That is why I write books. I have found books to be perfect vehicles to teach people I am unable to work with on a one-to-one basis.

One might ask, "Just how much can I learn from a book?" Although it's not the same as having a trainer in the room with you, it is a great alternative for when a trainer is just not possible. I have received hundreds of stories of people who bought my books and used them to produce wonderful results. Recently, I received word of a 60-year-old man who used my book, *Body Mastery*, to get into shape after suffering a life-threatening heart attack. As of his last check-up, his doctor had given him a clean bill of health and had taken him off all medications.

Another success story that sticks in my mind is the story of another man who read *Body Mastery*. He was the vice president of a construction company. He had been unhappy for quite some time with his situation. He simply had outgrown working for somebody else. He knew his ideas were great, and he wanted to control his own destiny. The thing that was holding him back was the courage to make the change. However, after mastering his body and getting himself into great shape, he developed the confidence to take the plunge. He said, "Getting my body in shape gave me the confidence to jump in and take the risk. After all, I had my health, I felt good about myself, so what if I didn't make it in business? It wouldn't be the end of the world."

There are also many weight loss success stories, as well as stories of people who have used my books to help them get in shape, increase their income, and overcome personal challenges.

Training Yourself contains everything you need to know to take charge physically, experience peak fitness, develop the body of your dreams, live a healthy lifestyle, sharpen your mental skills, and become a peak performer and high achiever. With *Training Yourself* you will learn how to become your own trainer and you will be able to pursue and reach your goals.

The book is divided into four parts:

Part One—General Fitness Training And More

In Part One I will discuss all the important elements for general fitness. Included are programs for the beginning, intermediate, and advanced levels. There are chapters on aerobic training, basics of weight training, performance nutrition, shape training for women, training and pregnancy, training for safe weight loss and safe weight gain, as well as on stretching and flexibility, overtraining and injuries, and the importance of supplements.

If you are just starting out, I recommend that you read Part One. It is loaded with valuable information, insights, training techniques, and exercise demonstration photographs.

Part Two—More Great Exercises for Shaping Up

Part Two contains my favorite training exercises for body parts. I am constantly asked, "What can I do about flabby arms, or a weak back, or a sagging rear end, or various other body areas? What exercises do you recommend? I need some special attention in this area."

In order to answer these questions, I have included a variety of exercises that you can incorporate into your training program to help you zero in on those challenge areas and keep your program fresh. You will learn the specific exercises that shape and develop the chest, back, shoulders, arms, abdominals, legs, and hips and thighs. These exercises are great for adding variety and giving your body that little extra attention that it may need to get into super shape.

Part Three—Training For Your Favorite Sport

Everyone agrees that a well-conditioned athlete is a better performer. Getting yourself into great shape is the best way to improve sports performance and prevent injuries, burnout, and fatigue. That is why Part Three is dedicated to training for your favorite sport. This section is comprised of specific training programs for three of the most popular adult sports: running, golf, and tennis. Each of these chapters contains my favorite training routines with the recommended sports-specific exercises.

Part Four—Getting Your Mind Into Your Training

Here is my favorite part of the book. This section is designated to help you develop the right mind-set and get your head into your training. Modern psychology has taught us that the mind leads the body—our minds produce thoughts, and thoughts govern our lives. Thoughts cause us to be who we are and act the way we do. Your body is in its present condition because, in a way, you thought it. Your thoughts actually were part of the blueprints that constructed it.

Most people make the mistake of treating exercise as a purely physical activity, figuring that all that is required to get into shape is physical exercise and a good diet. The mind, however, plays a critical role in the outcome, as in all great accomplishments. People who attempt training without building the correct mind-set don't succeed. They are the ones you see play the yo-yo game. If you want to achieve long-term success, the mental strategies covered in this section are a must. I cannot emphasize enough the importance of implementing them into your training program.

These chapters contain information on developing a training ethic, thinking big, taking responsibility, adjusting your attitude, setting goals for your body, getting the most out of each training session, and supercharging your motivation. This section contains the tools that will empower you to turn from dreamer into achiever!

How To Use This Book

You may be haunted by doubts about how much you can really change your body. Or you may lack confidence in your ability to succeed at such a challenging task. Take a minute and look at my before and after pictures on this page. I think you'll see that it is truly possible to change your body. Obviously, I am very qualified to tell you that you can indeed change your body. I always tell my clients, "You can do amazing things. As a matter of fact, you can do a lot more than you can't do." In other words, there are very few limits. While you can't alter the basic bone structure of your body, training will give your body more appeal, shape, definition, and eye-pleasing symmetry.

There are, however, some secrets that you must learn. Secrets such as developing and implementing the right training program, following the right diet, developing the right mind-set. Consider this book a resource guide, a complete encyclopedia of information for shaping up your body and mind. Each chapter in the book is self-contained and complete. You do not have to read the book from cover to cover to successfully use it. Like an encyclopedia, you can easily and quickly research the

Kris, age 20 (weighing 250 lbs.)

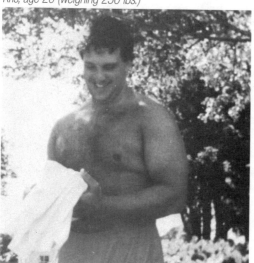

Kris, age 35 (weighing 185 lbs.)

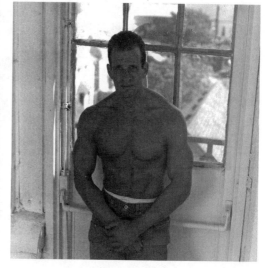

information of interest. For example, if your goal is to lose weight, turn to Chapter Thirteen and follow the "Safe Weight Loss Training Program." If your goal is to gain weight, turn to Chapter Fourteen and follow the "Fat Free Weight Gain Training Program." Look up information on topics such as nutrition, anatomy, burnout, fatigue, overtraining, injuries, etc. to help you reach your physical goals

Something You Should Know Before You Continue
If you like page after page of theories, statistics, and conclusions drawn from laboratory experiments, this book is not for you. What you are about to read is based on personal experience, including 21 years of training myself and the many years I have worked one-to-one with clients.

When I first picked up a dumbbell at age 14, I couldn't have imagined that I would be conducting a real-life experiment on the long-term effects of training and fitness. Looking back, I guess you could say I was a guinea pig for training longevity. But then you couldn't have convinced me that I would someday become a positive example of the long-term effects of training. What I learned out there in the real world—by doing—is what you are going to learn in this book. The information was gained from the laboratory of life, the school of hard knocks!

During a recent training session, a client asked me a very important question. He said, "How do some health care professionals—trainers, nutritionists, etc.—get away with being overweight and out of shape? How do they justify it? How can they tell others they need to take care of their health when they obviously don't do it themselves?" I answered, "It's my personal belief that it's not good enough to just give the message. I believe you have to be the message." It's a great feeling for me to be able to speak from that perspective. I am very proud to say, what you are about to read, I am.

New Light On A Worn-Out Topic
Perhaps the most exciting thing about this book is that it sheds new light on an old, worn-out topic: diet and exercise. It's ho-hum to fire yourself up to go to the gym to shed a few pounds for swimsuit season. It's pretty hard to get yourself out of bed at 6 a.m. to jog around the block hoping to lower your cholesterol a few points. But it's invigorating to spring into the gym to train to make more money, catapult yourself up the career ladder, produce a gold record, or start your own business!

There are many reasons to become involved in a fitness program: to look better, to be healthier, to reduce stress in your life, to win a mate, to get stronger—the list could go on. But I believe it's best to adopt the philosophy of training for self-development—training to become a better person. This is an approach that will take you far beyond looking good for your class reunion.

Training for self-development blends physical fitness with mental and emotional development. The goal is always to develop the whole person—body and mind. Where the mind goes, the body will follow. Think about what that will do for your body. Think about what that will do for your life!

Through the pages of this book, I have the privilege of passing these success secrets to you so you too can adopt them and use them to achieve your dreams and desires. This book encompasses some of the most powerful body-, mind-, and life-changing ideas known. To put it simply, you are about to discover and learn principles and practices that will not only dramatically change your physical world but will transform your entire life for the better. The secrets that you'll learn in the pages of this book will give you the power to turn your wishes into reality. It will teach you how to train yourself to reach levels of personal excellence that you never thought you could reach!

Chapter 2
Setting Up A Successful Training Program

Few people really understand the complexity of training. For most, getting started on a training program means joining a gym and copying a friend's workout program. When I custom-design a training program for a client, they are often amazed at just how much goes into formulating it.

Webster's Dictionary defines "training" as a means to instruct or condition to some manner of behavior or performance. "Program" is described as the organized effort to achieve a goal by stages or a set of logical steps to solve a problem. So your training program could be thought of as an organized effort of logical steps of instruction and conditioning that will help you to produce the behavior, performance, and results that you desire.

A successful training program must have a well-developed plan, centered around activities and exercises that are conducive to the ultimate goal. So just as an Olympic athlete needs to develop a training program to get into the best shape possible to compete in this world event, so too must you develop a program that will sharpen your skills to reach your goals—whatever they may be.

Careful attention must be given to the formulation of your training program. It's not just an exercise, a mindless activity, or pure recreation. A good training program should be thought of as self-development—activities that sharpen your skills to become the best you can be.

Training Is a Time for Discovery
In training you will learn much about yourself. You will go beyond your former boundaries, face challenges, overcome fears and weaknesses, and, at the same time,

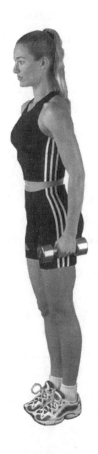

build new strengths. Your training program will stimulate positive feelings and emotions—the fuel you need to actively pursue all of your goals.

There are many secrets to formulating a successful training program. The first is that it is unique to you. Your training program is yours. Don't expect to train in exactly the same way as your friends. Developing your training program is going to involve your efforts. It requires self-study, personal assessment, and careful calculation, as well as commitment, persistence, and consistency.

Once you've decided that you are going to start a training program, you will need to put together an action plan—a system or an organized way of accomplishing your goals. It will require a series of practices or training sessions, grouped together and practiced consistently in order for you to obtain the results you desire.

And notice throughout this book I use the word "train" or "training." To me training stimulates positive physical and mental growth. A "workout" implies drudgery and is usually something not engaged in with enthusiasm. So every time you start to say, "I gotta go work out" with a long sigh—stop yourself and switch your choice of words and your tone to reflect enthusiasm. "I'm going to go train!"

There's a universal law that states what you sow, so shall you reap. This literally means that you get back exactly what you put out. For instance, if you approach your training sessions with enthusiasm, you will gain energy. If you approach your training sessions with dread and a feeling that you "should" go "work out," you will very likely leave the gym feeling depleted of energy.

The Structure Of Your Training Program

There are many different ways to train, as well as many different opinions and theories on what makes a good training program. It's very easy to get frustrated, confused, and misled.

Each month the in-vogue fitness magazines present different training programs and exercises which very often leave the reader wondering which way is right. Again, it's important to remember that there are many different ways and reasons to train and no one way is right over another. What is correct depends on your goals and your activities.

Some experts are going to tell you to lift weights three times a week, others twice a week. Some are going to tell you to eat a high carbohydrate diet; others will tell you to keep your carbohydrate intake low. I have found that there is really no universal "right way" to train. The only right way is the one that works for you and that you feel comfortable with. The way you determine which way is right for you is to experiment and try different routines and exercises, then judge the results. This is done by listening to your inner voice—tapping into how your body feels and responds to a particular training program. You need to judge it by the results you get. Then you need to change it if it just doesn't feel right or if it's not working. Your body ultimately knows best.

There are five very important factors that need to be considered in every training program:

1. Personal Training Philosophy
2. Individual Characteristics
3. Goals
4. Lifestyle
5. Specific Needs

Personal Training Philosophy

Your Personal Training Philosophy could be defined as your current and evolving beliefs about training in general. It's your basic theory of training. As I mentioned in Chapter One, my personal training philosophy centers around training for self-development. Again, that means not only training to get into shape but to become a better person all the way around—a peak performer in all areas of life. This means that I am training to get into fantastic shape, and I am also training to become a better author, father, employer, husband, and citizen. This is a good philosophy because it extends your motivation and drive to continue training outside of your immediate goals. Those who adopt this philosophy will continue to train forever--as long as the desire to improve themselves remains. Those who don't usually stop training when they get in shape.

Individual Characteristics

Another very important factor relating to the success of your training program is your Individual Characteristics. As human beings we were all created differently. You are unique. So it makes sense then that no one generic training program is going to work best for each of us. The best training program is the one that has been custom molded to fit your individual characteristics and needs. This is accomplished by taking an inventory of your personal characteristics and personal situations. However, this is not as hard as it sounds. You can simply begin with a generic training program like the ones in this book, and as you experiment with it you can adjust it to fit your needs. A generic exercise program can't take into consideration your personal characteristics, individual ability, goals, level of experience, motivation, or resources. The following are individual characteristics for you to keep in mind.

1. Body Type

It is extremely important to get an idea of your body type in order to ensure that you are participating in the correct type of workout that will provide you with the best results. When I set up a training program for a client, I take their body type into consideration. If they are short and stocky, I know that they will most likely find it relatively easy to put on muscle mass. So I will recommend that they do a variety of basic movements but also a variety of shaping movements. This allows them to develop proportionately, well-shaped muscles instead of just thick, bulky ones. I move them through their workouts with the least amount of rest time between sets and reps, and I pay close attention to their diet.

The key is to recognize your body type and then apply the right training program. Learning and understanding your body type can save you a lot of wasted time and frustration. Although certain principles of training are the same for all body types, the way in which you set up your program and the techniques you adopt can make a profound difference depending on what type of body you were given at birth.

You can even change your body type to some degree. Look at the pictures on page 11. In the picture on the left, weighing 250 pounds, I look very large and bulky. On the right, I now look streamlined, well-defined, and in shape. By discovering your body type and applying these training programs for your body, you could achieve fantastic results.

2. Current Level Of Fitness

Your current level of fitness is a critical element you must consider when designing your program. I frequently see people get their ambitions smashed by setting their sights too high and going at it too hard and too quickly, especially when they are terribly out of shape. This usually results in burnout, injury, and loss of motivation to train. What is your current condition?

3. Training Experience

Your training experience is a very important factor of consideration; however, it is not a limiting factor. How much training experience do you have? More times than not, clients who come to me with no prior experience wind up being the most successful. So don't fret over lack of experience. Remember this—when I first started weight training, I didn't even know the difference between a dumbbell and a weight machine.

5. Physical Energy

How much "fuel" do you have to dedicate to your training? All of us have different energy levels. Some have high levels, some low. There are many things that affect your energy level. In the following chapters you will learn how to increase your energy as well as how to avoid things that zap your energy. Remember: everything in life requires energy—whether you're climbing the corporate ladder, building your business, or raising your kids. Energy production will be very important to you, both now and in the future.

6. Motivation Level

Your motivation level is as unique as your body type. All of us are motivated differently and at different levels or degrees. Obviously someone with a higher level of motivation is going to need a more stimulating training program. It's important that you match your training program appropriately to your level of motivation. If not you'll have a mismatch that will create varying degrees of frustration and a lack of interest. You will need to continually work to develop your motivation. It's not something that we are born with.

Goals

You need to be able to define and have a clear understanding of your goals and objectives. Goals are the "what" you want to accomplish. You will need to spend some time seriously thinking about what you really want to accomplish in your training program. And you need to be more specific than just saying you want to start to exercise or get in shape. Your goals need to be more clear and more specific, such as "I want to gain 10 pounds of muscle." Or, "I want to decrease my body fat percent by one tenth."

At first, you may have a hard time identifying your specific goals, but with practice it will become easier and your goals will become more clear.

Lifestyles

Balance and good decision making are also important factors to a successful training program. Training should not throw your life out of balance. It should fit into your lifestyle relatively comfortably. While there may be some sacrifices to make and some bad habits to shed, your training program should enhance your life.

An unbalanced approach to training always leads to burnout, fatigue, and overtraining. Many people jump into a training program full of enthusiasm, adopting a more-is-better attitude. While they may achieve some quick results, as times goes on very few of these people continue training at all.

Remember the tale of the tortoise and the hare—slow and steady wins the race.

Specific Needs

There are many important decisions you need to make before beginning your training program, as well as many decisions you will need to make as you progress through your training. All decisions are important, regardless of their size and magnitude. You need to ask yourself:

* Where am I going to train—at the office, the club, home?
* What type of training program do I want to use?
* When am I going to train?
* Am I going to need a training partner?
* Do I need a trainer or a coach?
* Can I obtain the information I need through books, tapes, and videos?

These are important considerations. I've seen many people make crucial mistakes with the decisions they make, like picking the wrong place to train or not getting the proper instruction.

The Complete Training Program

In order for a training program to be totally effective, it should be complete. A complete training program should center around six key areas:

* Mental training exercises
* Aerobic (cardiovascular) exercises
* Weight training exercises
* Good nutrition practices
* Attention to recovery
* A system of checks and balances

Mental Training

Mental training is what I refer to as "brain building." These are mental exercises like goal setting, visualization, and self-talk. These exercise are designed to strengthen, tone, and develop your intellectual muscles. Successful training is not just the result of physical activity. Where the mind goes the body will follow. In Part Four, I will introduce you to many brain-building exercises that will help you train in a more focused manner, as well as increase your motivation, desire, and commitment.

Aerobic (Cardiovascular) Exercise

Proper conditioning of the cardiovascular system (heart, lungs, circulatory system) is important in your overall health and well-being. It is a vital ingredient to get your body in tip-top shape and in good working order.

There are a wide range of exercises, activities, and routines designed to develop and condition your cardiovascular system. These include walking, jogging, running, stair climbing, stationary biking, rowing, cross-country skiing, aerobic classes, and weight training.

Remember, you will have unique cardiovascular training needs. Training intensity, routines, and activities will ultimately be determined by your goals and current fitness level. Chapter Four will give you in-depth instruction on how to develop your own aerobic training program. Further instruction for specific sports will be addressed in the following chapters.

Weight Training

Weight training or resistance training is by far the best and most practical way to strengthen, tone, shape, and mold body muscles. For the purposes of this book, resistance training centers around weight training exercises: free weights (dumbbells and barbells) and weight machines.

The goals of weight training are to increase and maintain strength, develop muscle mass, shape, tone, and increase muscular endurance. Adopting the style of weight training that I am teaching will not make you a 300-pound, bulked-out sumo wrestler. My style of weight training will help you develop an in-shape body and better conditioning.

In the chapters that follow, you will be given advice on how to design your program at different training levels. There will be information on weight training for general fitness and sports. Stretching, lifting techniques, sets, reps, and cool-downs will also be discussed.

And before you can effectively use weights to mold and shape your muscles, you must know where to look for the muscles. I have included basic anatomy illustrations in Chapter Three. However, with over 600 muscles in the body, you can be sure that I'm not going to discuss every muscle. I'll give you just the information that you need to be successful with your training.

Nutrition

Good nutritional practices will probably determine between 60 and 80 percent of your overall training success. This area is often neglected and overlooked by people who train for fitness and health.

Whether your goal is to lose, gain, or maintain weight, to increase strength, enhance muscle tone, and/or to increase stamina and endurance, you will want to get an in-depth understanding of nutrition. Your eating habits affect your health, appearance, performance, moods, and energy levels.

In Chapter Seven, we examine important nutritional topics such as when to eat, what to eat, why to eat, and how to eat. We'll look at supplements, suggested foods, meal schedules, food journals, shortcuts, as well as secrets and tips for maintaining good nutritional practices. To provide your body with the nutrients it needs to develop, perform at its best, and recover from training and everyday stresses means eating the right combination of foods along with adopting a good supplementation program.

This doesn't mean you will never be able to eat out again. You'll still be able to go to your favorite restaurant. You may, however, find yourself choosing energy producing foods, while your companions opt for energy draining fries and greasy burgers.

Recovery

Like nutrition, too often the recovery stage of a training program is overlooked and seldom discussed. But recovery is just as important as the actual training session.

Because of the mental and physical demands of training, it's very important place special importance on recovery. In weight training, the muscles do not increase in size (hypertrophy) until after they have thoroughly recovered from your preceding workout. Muscles grow during the resting phase of training, not during the actual lifting. I have a training equation that I follow:

Intelligent Training + Nutrition + Rest = Results

Physical training is an important part of your program, but overtraining is often the cause of failure. Training too hard, too long, and too often—without the proper attention to recovery—is going to diminish the results you get, and perhaps even set you up for injury and burnout.

Intelligent training means getting the most from the least amount of effort. However, you must train with intensity and focus. Merely going through the motions will get you nowhere. And you must eat nutritious foods for your body to recover.

Rest is also a vital part of the recovery process. We all know that the body requires rest to perform at its best. This includes adequate sleep and enough relaxation time during our waking hours to bring about a state of physical and mental refreshment. This too is individualized. Some people can get by with seven or eight hours sleep; others need 10 or 12.

Training places many demands on you physically and mentally. In order to be successful with your program you need to figure into your training schedule time off, sleep, recreation, stress managements, rest periods, and layoffs. In the following chapter I make recommendations for your training program that will include attention to recovery. Take these seriously.

System Of Checks And Balances

It's pretty hard to stick to something if the effort you are investing isn't giving you a payoff, or you don't feel like you're making any progress.

It is extremely important that you set up a system of checks and balances to keep track of your progress. It is essential that you give yourself this kind of feedback, because if you don't you will be less likely to stick with the program.

Checks and balances fall into two categories—informal and scientific. For general fitness most people rely on the informal methods to gauge their progress. These include photographs, videotaping, tape measures, and scales. They're easy to use and require little time and effort.

If you're more technical, there are more scientific methods for testing your body's response to your training program. These include muscular fitness tests, cardiovascular fitness tests, and body composition analysis. These offer a more precise, scientific measurement of your progress and seem to appeal to people who are more statistically minded and like cold, hard facts.

Your training program should become a very special part of your life. For the best results, view it as a lifelong commitment to self-development, growth, and advancement in all areas of your life. A training session should be thought of as a chapter in the book of your life. It's not just a workout. It's a sacred time that you invest today to make yourself better in the future. There's no question that physical fitness affects your total well-being. It spills over directly into every nook and cranny of your existence. Treat your training program—and in essence your body—with the importance and respect that it deserves.

Chapter 3
Training Anatomy

The Wonder Machine
Have you ever really thought about all the things your body does in a 24-hour period? It can be mind-boggling. Your body has hundreds of intricately devised cells, muscles, and bones (not to mention the organs), which synchronically work together to get you through your day. And the best thing about your body and its functions is that you don't have to think about it at all—that is, unless you want it to perform even better.

The Parts
Getting started on a training program requires that you learn about your body. Specifically, we are concerned with two things:

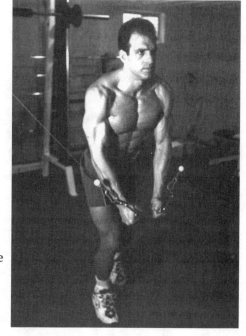

* The muscles of the body—how they work, where they are, and what they do
* Your cardiovascular system (heart, lungs, and circulatory system)—how it works, what its function is during exercise

However, in the first stages of training, it is not necessary that you dissect a cadaver and study and memorize all of the over 600 muscles in the body. In fact, you really don't have to know more than the basic muscle groups and be able to locate them on your body. As you advance with your training, you may want to increase your knowledge further and learn more.

The Muscles Of The Machine
For training purposes, the body can be divided into six groups: chest, back, shoulders, arms, midsection, and lower body.

The Chest

The pectoral consists of two parts—the clavicular (upper) portion and the sternal (lower) portion. The upper part is attached to the clavicle (collarbone). Along the midbody line, it attaches to the sternum (breastbone) and to the cartilage of several ribs. The largest mass of the pectoral starts at the upper arm bone (humerus), and is fastened at a point under and just above where the deltoids attach to the humerus. The pectorals spread out like a fan and cover the rib cage like armor plates.

Attached to the rib cage in the center and across to the shoulder, this muscle lets you perform such motions as pitching a ball underhanded, doing a wide arm bench press, or twisting a cap off a bottle.

The Back

The flat triangular muscle that extends out and down from the neck and down between the shoulder blades is the trapezius. The primary function of the trapezius is to raise the shoulder girdle.

The latissimus dorsi (lats) are the large triangular muscles that extend from under the shoulders down to the small of the back on both sides. Their primary function is to pull the shoulders downward.

The spinal erectors, composed of several muscles in the lower back that guard the nerve channels, work to hold the spine erect, straighten the spine from a position with the torso flexed completely forward, and help to arch the lower and middle back.

The Shoulder

The deltoids are versatile muscles that move the arm forward, backward, to the side, up, and around. The deltoids have three distinct lobes of muscle called "heads" that enable this movement: the anterior head (the muscle in the front), the medial head (the muscle on the side), and the posterior head (the muscle in the rear).

The Arms

The bicep (biceps brachii) is a two-headed muscle with its point of origin under the deltoid and its point of insertion below the elbow. There are two muscle groups located at the front of the upper arm that contract to flex the arm fully from a straight position. The smallest of these muscles is called the brachialis, a thin band of muscle between the biceps and triceps. The brachialis muscle runs only about halfway up the humerus bone above the elbow.

The biceps are much larger in mass than the brachialis muscles and are the primary muscle group responsible for bending the arm. With an origin near the shoulder joint and insertions on the forearm bones, the biceps bend the arm from a straight position. The secondary function of the biceps is to supinate the hand. The biceps make up about 35 percent of the arm mass.

The tricep (triceps brachii), a three-headed muscle that attaches under the deltoid and below the elbow, works in opposition to the biceps to straighten the arm and supinate (twist upward) the wrist. The triceps are larger than the biceps and make up about three-quarters of the upper arm.

The forearm is composed of a variety of muscles on the outside and inside of the lower arm that control the actions of the hand and wrist. The forearm flexor muscles curl the palm down and forward; the forearm extensor muscles curl the knuckles back and up.

The Midsection

The visual center of the body—the abdomen—is composed of the rectus abdominis, the external obliques, and the intercostals. The abdominals have a relatively simple function. They pull your upper body (rib cage) and lower body (pelvis) toward each other, and they contribute to keeping your internal organs in place.

The rectus abdominis is a long muscle extending along the length of the ventral aspect of the abdomen. This muscle originates in the area of the pubis and inserts into the cartilage of the fifth, sixth, and seventh ribs. The basic function of the rectus abdominis is to support the spinal column and draw the sternum toward the pelvis.

The external obliques (obliques externus abdominis) are the muscles at each side of the torso (commonly referred to as the handles). They are attached to the lower eight ribs and insert at the sides of the pelvis. The basic function of the external obliques is to flex and rotate the spinal column.

The intercostals are two thin planes of muscles and tendon fibers occupying the spaces between the ribs. The intercoastals lift the ribs and draw them together.

The Lower Body

The lower body is made up of more than 200 muscles. The majority of these muscles are located in the thighs, hips, and buttocks. Rather than trying to explain the development of every one of these muscles, we will focus on the development of the legs and buttocks. We'll also examine the main muscle groups and the function in each one.

The primary muscles of the buttocks are the gluteus maximus and the gluteus medius. The gluteus maximus contracts to help straighten the legs and torso from a completely or partially flexed position.

The thighs are among the largest muscles in the human body. The main thigh muscles are the quadricepts and the hamstrings.

The quadriceps contract to straighten the leg from a fully or partially bent position. The quadriceps are composed of four muscles at the front of the thigh—rectus femoris, vastus intermedius, vastus medialis, and vastus lateralis.

The hamstrings, the primary muscle group at the back of the thigh is the biceps femoris, are often called the leg biceps. This muscle group contracts to bend the leg fully from a straight or partially bent position.

The primary muscles of the calves are the soleus, gastrocnemius, and the tibialis anterior. The soleus is the larger and deeper of the calf muscles and originates from both the fibula and the tibia. Its basic function is to flex the foot. The gastrocnemius has two heads, one originating from the lateral aspect and the other from the medial of the lower femur. Both heads join to overlay the soleus and join with and insert into the Achilles tendon which inserts into the heel bone. The basic function of the gastrocnemius is to flex the foot. The tibialis anterior runs up the front of the lower leg alongside the shinbone. Its basic function is to flex the foot.

The Cardiovascular/Aerobic Parts Of The Human Machine

Science tells us the primary function of the cardiovascular system is to deliver blood to active tissues. This includes the delivery of oxygen and nutrients and the removal of metabolic waste products. During prolonged bouts of exercise your cardiovascular system also maintains your body temperature so you won't overheat. The cardiovascular system is composed of lungs, blood vessels, heart, arteries, capillaries, and veins.

Being successful with any training program is going to require that you learn the basic anatomy outlined in this chapter. Knowing what the muscles do, where they are located, and their primary function during training is necessary to correctly follow and apply any specific training program.

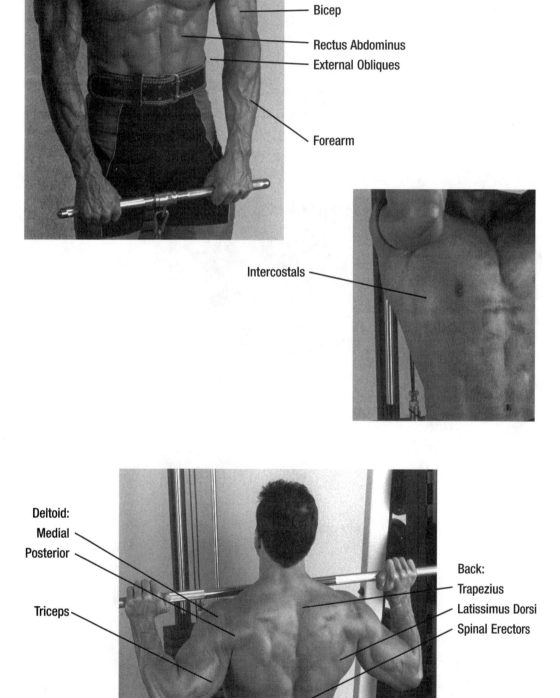

TRAINING ANATOMY

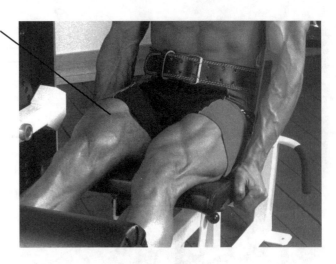

Quadriceps:
(Rectus Femoris
Vastus Intermedius
Vastus Medialis
Vastus Lateralis)

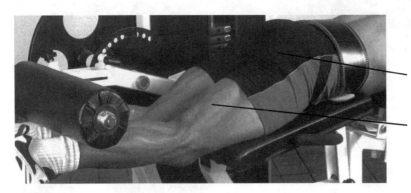

Gluteus Maximus

Hamstring

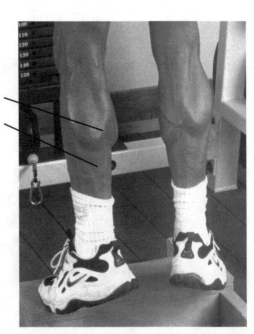

Calves:
Gastrocnemius
Soleus

Chapter 4
Aerobic Training

If you want to get into great shape, control your weight, improve performance, and become fit and healthy, then you will want to include aerobic (cardiovascular) exercise in your training program.

A Quick Lesson In Cardiovascular Training

Cardiovascular training conditions the heart, lungs, and circulatory system. It also helps to control body weight. Your heart is the most important muscle in your body. It is a muscular pump, about the size of your fist, that beats nonstop every minute of your life, sending about 2,000 gallons of blood through your body every day.

If you want to create a strong, healthy, and in-shape body that can perform at its best, you must not neglect your cardiovascular training. Looking great on the outside means little if your heart and lungs are not functioning properly on the inside. Exercises that force you to elevate your heart rate are referred to as aerobic exercise because they allow you to breath at a steady, continuous pace as you perform them. Walking, jogging, stair climbing, treadmilling, stationary biking, rowing, cross-country skiing, doing aerobics, and many competitive sports all exercise the cardiovascular system.

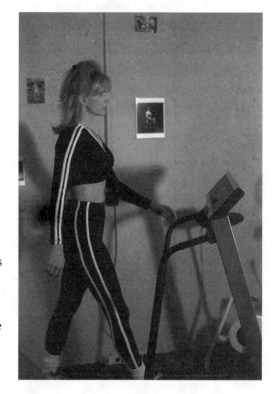

Your Cardiovascular System

Science tells us that the major function of the cardiovascular system during exercise is to deliver blood to active tissues. This includes the delivery of oxygen and nutrients and the removal of the metabolic waste products. If you exercise long enough, your cardiovascular system will also maintain your body temperature so that you won't overheat.

Anaerobic activities use the large muscle groups, but at high intensities that exceed the body's capacity to use oxygen to supply energy. This creates an oxygen deficit by using energy produced without oxygen. Anaerobic exercise (weight lifting) eventually builds up enough of an oxygen deficit to force the exerciser to terminate the exercise session quickly. That is why you eventually run out of gas and have to stop when lifting weights.

For any training program to be complete, you should consider three primary goals for exercising the cardiovascular system.

>1. Increase the capacity of the cardiovascular system
>2. Use the cardiovascular system to prolong periods of exercise in order to promote fat burning if you're trying to maintain weight or lose weight
>3. Help in developing muscle mass, strength, muscle toning, and muscular endurance and recovery

Your number one goal of cardiovascular exercise should be to condition the cardiovascular system. You want to increase the capacity of your respiratory system—the lungs and blood vessels—and your circulatory system—heart, arteries, capillaries, and veins—in order to supply oxygen and nutrients to your muscles' cells so that you can sustain physical activity for at least 30 continuous minutes. This is the minimum amount of time scientists tell us we need to exercise in order to maintain cardiovascular fitness.

Finding Your Target

You will need to focus on aerobic activities and exercise that permit you to get into the aerobic training zone, sometimes called the target zone. These exercises, although strenuous, are rhythmic, and performed in a range of intensity that allows you to safely elevate your heart rate for cardiovascular benefit. You can accomplish this by walking, jogging, or using the treadmill. I like to use a heart monitor to check my heart rate and to see if I'm in the proper range for my training program.

The aerobic training zone is estimated to be between 60 and 85 percent of your maximum heart rate. If you're a beginner, simply subtract your age from 220, then multiply by 60 percent. If you are at an

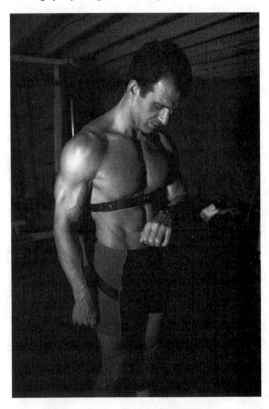

intermediate fitness level, subtract your age from 220 and multiply by 70 percent. If you're at an advanced level, subtract your age from 220 and multiply by 85 percent. The figure you arrive at represents the number of times your heart needs to beat per minute to derive the most cardiovascular benefit.

To reach the aerobic training zone, you need to engage in an aerobic workout consisting of a five- to ten-minute warm-up, followed by 20 minutes of aerobic training, and ending with a five- to ten-minute cool down. The warm-up increases your heart rate gradually, which prepares your muscular and circulatory systems for the upcoming training period. A good warm-up also helps prevent injuries to muscles, ligaments, and joints. The training period should last 20 to 30 minutes to keep your heart rate elevated in your training zone. The cool down allows your muscular and circulatory system to return to normal levels. A proper cool down will help to prevent dizziness, faintness, or nausea. It's important to train your cardiovascular system three times a week with no more than two days between training sessions to achieve a reasonable cardiovascular fitness level.

The Fat Burning Training Zone

Training at a lower intensity for longer periods of time has proven to be an effective way to burn body fat. You can enhance the burning of unwanted body fat by lowering the intensity of aerobic exercise to the 50 to 65 percent range of your maximum heart rate, and extending the time and frequency of your training sessions.

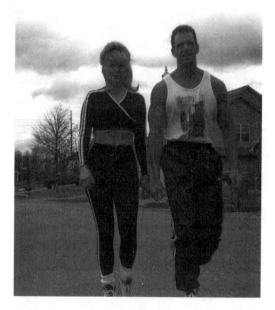

Exercises should be of moderate intensity, like slow jogging.

You can compute your fat burning training zone by using the same formula for the aerobic training zone. The training routine is also similar. It should consist of a five- to ten-minute warm-up, followed by 45 to 60 minutes of low intensity exercise, and end with five to ten minutes of cool down. You should also increase the number of training sessions to four or five per week.

Anaerobic Training Zone

I have learned that anaerobic training can compliment aerobic and fat burning for individuals at advanced levels of training. This type of training is excellent for increasing muscle mass, definition, tone, increasing stamina, power, speed, endurance, and strength—all of which are important in developing a totally conditioned body. This type of exercise is extremely effective for developing the hips, thighs, hamstrings, and calves.

In order to reach your anaerobic training zone, you elevate the intensity of exercise to reach 85 to 100 percent of your maximum heart rate.

This is not something I recommend for any beginner. Anaerobic exercises can be added to your training program as you progress in your fitness level. I like to use wind sprints for anaerobic training. I started with five to ten minutes of warm-up jogging, followed by a series of four 40-yard sprints. Then I move up to four 50-yard sprints, followed by two 70-yard sprints. I finished with one 100-yard sprint then cool down with a slow jog for five to ten minutes.

There are many different forms of cardiovascular/aerobic exercise. Yet all are not created equal. Some are better suited for specific training goals. Treadmill walking tends to be a great choice for burning body fat. Jogging is best for building aerobic conditioning, and wind sprints are the best for anaerobic training. I recommend that you incorporate a variety of exercises into your training program.

The following is a partial list of many aerobic training options that I feel bring the most success since they can easily fit into the busiest lifestyle.

Treadmills—I recommend the treadmill first because it is a weight-bearing exercise. It's also the most natural, which makes it the easiest to learn. The treadmill is also my first recommendation for fat burning. It forces you to keep a steady pace and stride. When people walk outside they have a tendency to slow down; traffic, neighbors, and dogs often force you to break stride.

Recumbent and Stationary Bikes—These are good because they are easy to use, easy on the body, and excellent for getting your heart rate up. They are also relatively inexpensive and can fit nicely into the corner of the family room.

Step Climbers—These are more challenging. They don't work the upper body the way the treadmill does. They also require more athletic ability and coordination than a bike or treadmill.

Good fat burning exercises include:

* Walking on the treadmill
* Jogging (slow pace) on the treadmill, street, or track
* Stationary biking — either upright or recumbent

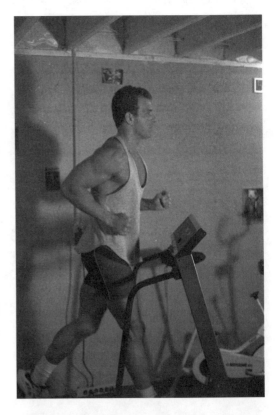

The Secrets Of Aerobics

Understand the different training zones and effectively apply them to your training goals

Get enough cardiovascular training to keep your heart and lungs in shape

Use the cardiovascular training split method consisting of warm-up, weights, cool down

Find exercises that you enjoy and that are relatively comfortable to perform

Change your exercises frequently

Vary the intensity, time, and length of your training sessions
Remember: A steady diet of the same exercise will eventually lead to mental and physical burnout

This type of exercise is high intensity and requires all out effort. You shouldn't rush to add this type of training into your routine until you have had several good months, and in some cases years, under your belt.

Anaerobic exercises are:

* Sprinting on the treadmill
* Wind Sprints at the track
* Hill climbing — out in nature or on the treadmill
* Stationary bike sprints
* Stadium bleacher running
* Interval running 220, 440

This is only a partial list of cardiovascular training exercises. These seem to be the ones that give the best results and that are most popular with my clients. Feel free to integrate any other cardiovascular exercises not mentioned here that allow you to reach your training goals into your program as well.

The Primary Focus

Remember, the number one goal for your aerobic training routine is to get your cardiovascular system in shape. Fat burning and anaerobic workouts can be implemented later as you get into better shape. You'll still be burning many calories and losing some body fat.

Strive to train aerobically two or three times a week for at least 20 minutes. You can increase the length of your workout and the number of workouts as your fitness level increases. Remember to listen to your body. If you get tired, dizzy, or faint, slow down or stop all together.

Aerobic/Weight Training Combinations

Optimally, you'll also be weight training as well. (We'll discuss weight training in the next chapter.) Here are my favorite combinations:

* Two training sessions a week—combining aerobics with weights
* Three training sessions a week—two aerobic/weight training sessions, and one solo aerobic session
* Three training sessions a week—combining aerobic and weight training

The Recreational Activity Myth

Too often people believe that the recreational activities such as golf, strolling around the neighborhood, beach volleyball, noncompetitive swimming, and shooting basketball produce cardiovascular benefits. These activities may be helpful in reducing stress and they may be fun, but they do not work the heart and lungs hard enough to produce aerobic, fat burning, or anaerobic benefits.

Recreational activities should be reserved for those times off you give your mind and body a rest from the stresses of the day, as well as your usual training program.

An Important Ingredient

Cardiovascular exercise is very important for general fitness training, health, and performance. It conditions and strengthens your heart and lungs, helps build endurance and stamina, and it is the best way to control weight and body fat. Cardiovascular exercises also promote muscular growth and aid recovery.

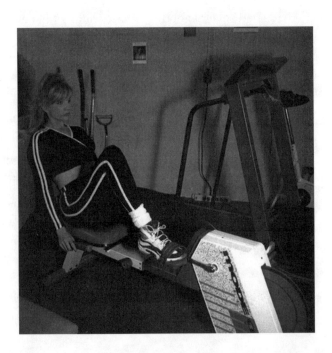

Chapter 5
The Basics Of Weight Training

It's important to know how and why weight training works before you pick up a weight. When muscles are subjected to resistance, they become more efficient, stronger, better toned. They develop increased blood flow and are less likely to ache or become injured. Exercising muscles properly counteracts muscular atrophy which occurs as we age. (The average man loses 50 percent of his muscle mass between 18 and 65 years of age.) Weight training exercises place a demand on the muscles, and as the muscles adapt to that demand, they become stronger and better able to sustain muscular activity.

Scientists are unable to tell us everything about resistance training; however, they do know that skeletal muscles are made up of thousands of muscle fibers and each fiber consists of many muscles strung end to end. When a muscle is subjected to resistance, it tears itself down and then rebuilds itself stronger than before to handle the resistance. That means when you subject your muscles to enough resistance to cause muscle fatigue, the muscles will be forced to rebuild themselves, becoming stronger, more toned, and better able to handle more stress.

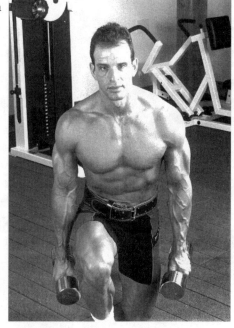

Your muscular system plays a major role in enabling you to perform the basic tasks of daily living; therefore, you must keep this system in proper working order so that you can keep on going comfortably and efficiently, whether you're striving for a gold medal or merely trying to stay on top of your studies and your social life. You keep your muscular system in top working order by adopting a good weight training program.

Three Forms Of Resistance Training

Weight training falls under the umbrella of resistance training—isometric, isotonic, and isokinetic.

Isometric resistance exercise is performed by resisting against an immovable object. For example, place your right hand on the top of your left hand with palm facing palm and then push them together. The

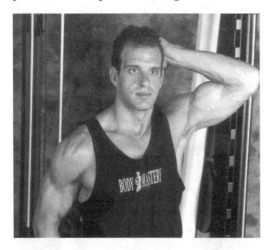

pressure produces an isometric contraction. Isometric exercises are most commonly used for rehabilitation or when conventional resistance training equipment is not available.

In isotonic resistance exercise there is resistance against equal tension, such as when lifting free weights or barbells. When you perform an isotonic exercise, such as a barbell arm curl, as you raise the barbell from the starting position to the ending position, the resistance throughout the plane of travel does not stay the same. Though the actual weight of the barbell doesn't change, the lift becomes either

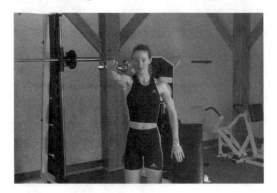

easier or harder as it progresses because of the body's natural mechanical advantage, called leverage. In isotonic lifting movements there is no accommodating resistance.

Isokinetic resistance exercises are most commonly performed on weight machines, such as those manufactured by Paramount and Cybex. With these types of machines, the accommodation resistance is varied by the use of cam, cables, pulleys, or the slide

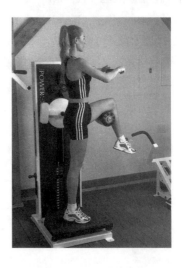

lever principle. These machines are designed to meet the body's natural strength curves by changing the amount of resistance throughout the movement. The end result is that the tension feels equal throughout the entire range of motion.

All three forms of resistant training are important in developing a completely balanced physique. I'll be recommending exercises from each of these three areas, but I'll be dropping the fancy technical terms for all but isometrics. Isotonic will be referred to as training with free weights; isokinetic as training with weight machines.

Weight Training Concepts

There are many different ways you could train with weights. For instance a powerlifter trains to get stronger to be able to lift the heaviest weight possible. A football player lifts weights to become bigger, stronger, and a faster, better athlete. The way a bodybuilder trains with weights, however, comes closest to the type of training you'll be undertaking by following the principles in this book. What I feel works best combines the focus of power lifting, sports training, and bodybuilding.

A bodybuilder lifts weights to build muscle mass, shape, tone, and enhance muscular development. The goal is to use weights to train the body for shape, definition, muscle mass, symmetry, proportion, strength, and power.

But before we actually get started with a program, it will be helpful to become familiar with the following definitions which I use frequently throughout this book.

Workout: a session of training. It can also be called a routine, program, or training schedule. A workout refers to the mental or written list of what you actually plan to do during your training session.

Exercise: each individual movement performed in your routine.

Repetition (or rep): one complete lifting movement. You perform one rep of an arm curl for example, by holding one free weight in each hand, arms down by your sides; then contract your arm muscles and raise the weights forward toward your shoulders. When the weights reach shoulder level, lower them back to the starting position at your sides. Reps are the number of completed lifting movements from start to finish.

Set: the number of reps completed in succession. For example if you perform ten complete reps of arm curls, rest for a moment, then perform ten more reps of arm curls, you will complete two full sets.

Rest interval: the recovery time between reps and sets. It usually varies anywhere from 30 seconds to five minutes depending on your condition and goals.

Weight: the actual pounds lifted or pressed.

Lifting motion: the plane of travel or the arc of movement. There are two planes of travel: the concentric or positive portion of movement and the eccentric or negative portion. The muscle shortens as it develops tension to overcome the resistance in the positive portion of a movement. During the negative portion, the muscle lengthens while developing tension. For instance, in the arm curl exercise, the downward part of the lift is the negative.

You'll want to be in control of the weight both in the positive and negative portions of the movements. This will allow you to achieve the full benefit from the exercise.

Feel: the sensation you get in your muscles as you perform an exercise. Tightness, firmness, swelling, and burning are all good reactions to resistance training.

The most important feeling is the pump, which is that swollen feeling you get in your muscles toward the end of a set. Muscle pump is caused by the rapid movement of blood into the muscles to remove fatigue toxins, while replacing supplies of fuel and oxygen. When you succeed at creating a good muscle pump, you have worked a muscle or muscle group optimally.

Burn is caused by a rapid build-up of fatigue toxins in a muscle, and it is a good indication that you have worked a muscle or muscle group optimally. Extending repetitions past the pump stage will produce a burn.

Three Important Goals Of Weight Training

It would be pointless to go into a gym and just lift weights without any rhyme or reason. Yet that's just what most people do. However, for complete physical development, you should consider the three important goals of weight training.

1. Increase Strength, Power, And Build Muscle Mass

Muscle mass is the size of each muscle or muscle group. The purpose of muscle is to generate force which requires strength, and strength is the foundation of the perfect body. The best way to develop strength is by lifting relatively heavy weights for a low number of reps.

Low Number of Reps + Heavy Weights = Strength

2. Tone Muscle

By toning, you will define, shape, and cause your muscles to become symmetrical. Muscle definition is the degree to which the muscle is developed. Often it is referred to as muscularity.

Shape refers to the pleasing pattern in the lines of a muscle. Proportion refers to the overall relationship between the size and the degree of development of all body parts. Symmetry is balance between the right and left sides of the body.

Medium Number of Reps + Medium Weights = Muscle Tone

3. Muscular Endurance

The ability of a muscle to produce force repeatedly over an extended period is considered muscular endurance. Movements that require maximum force, such as weight training, quickly deplete energy stores, and if you are not accustomed to these movements, you will quickly grow weak, feeling like you ran into a wall. Developing muscular endurance is very important because it enables you to complete more reps.

High Number of Reps + Light Weights = Muscular Endurance

Proper attention to developing strength, toning muscles, and increasing muscular endurance will encourage complete body development, give you the healthiest results, and get you into the best shape.

Chapter 6
The Basics of Nutrition

If you were to ask me what is the biggest mistake that I see people make in training, my answer would be nutrition. As I told my client one day when we were training, you can out eat any exercise program. By developing good nutritional habits, you will be able to increase physical energy, become more mentally clear, and improve your physical appearance.

Nutrients

Ultimately, you are responsible for everything that goes into your mouth. You can't push the responsibility onto your restaurant chefs or spouse. This means you need to:

* Learn the basic principles of nutrition
* Get an understanding of how foods affect your body
* Learn how to eat correctly and effectively

It is estimated that there are approximately 50 nutrients in food that are essential for the body's growth, maintenance, and repair. These are found in carbohydrates, proteins, and fats which provide the body with energy. They are also found in vitamins, minerals, and water, which are essential for your body to function in peak performance. If your body is deficient in even one of these components, you can become fatigued, become ill, even gain weight.

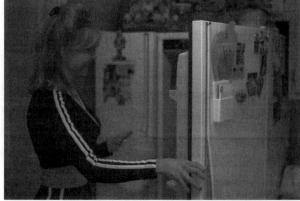

Carbohydrates

Simple and complex carbohydrates are a primary source of fuel for your body. Your body does not require a lot of simple carbohydrates, such as honey, sucrose, and table sugar. Simple carbohydrates cause a dramatic rise in blood sugar level creating an overproduction of insulin. Not good. Too much insulin takes too much sugar out of the bloodstream and causes you to feel tired and weak. It may also create an increase in fat deposition. On the other hand, complex carbohydrates, such as grains, pasta, potatoes, and other vegetables are broken down more slowly in the digestive system causing a more gradual increase in blood sugar level. The result is that you have more productive energy for a longer period. To fuel your body properly, you should eat mostly complex carbohydrates and avoid the simple carbohydrates.

Proteins

Proteins are essential for the growth and maintenance of all body tissue. They serve as a major source of building material for muscle, blood, skin, hair and nails, and for the internal organs, primarily the heart and brain. They also produce hormones that regulate a host of bodily functions, including growth, metabolic rates, sexual development, and antibodies that combat foreign substances in the body. During digestion, protein is broken down into simpler units called amino acids. In this state, amino acids enter a pool where they are stored for the body to draw upon when it needs new protein.

You get "good" protein from eggs, milk, chicken, and turkey, and "bad" protein from fatty red meats. With the exception of water, your body contains more protein than any other substance.

Complete And Incomplete Proteins

Just as all carbohydrates are not created equal, neither are protein foods. Therefore, you need to pay particular attention to the protein sources. There are incomplete and complete sources of protein. Incomplete protein sources are those foods that don't provide a good essential amino acid balance, such as fruits and vegetables. Complete protein sources are most meats and dairy products.

Fats

Fats are a secondary source of energy. Contrary to popular opinion, you should not eliminate fats completely from your diet because some fats are good for you. After your body has depleted all of the available stored muscle glycogen, it calls on fats to supply needed energy. Furthermore, fats carry and absorb the fat soluble vitamins A, D, E, and K. Fats supply the body with energy during periods of inactivity and during aerobic exercises. It surrounds and protects vital organs such as the kidneys, heart and liver. And finally, fat provides a blanket for preserving heat in the body.

Sodium

Sodium is necessary because it helps in transmitting nerve impulses. Too little sodium in your diet could cause severe cramping and weakness. But don't run over and pick up the salt shaker! It's easy to overdose on sodium in this country. The typical American diet contains more than ten times the minimum requirement of salt. That means it is highly unlikely that you are now, or will in the near future, become sodium deficient.

Most experts recommend 2,500-3,000 milligrams of sodium per day. A lunch of chips or fries, cheeseburger with condiments, commercial size pickle and flavored milk shake contains approximately 3,500 milligrams of sodium. That means that most people use up their allotted daily sodium intake in one meal!

If you eat good food in its most natural state, you will get an adequate supply of sodium without ever having to reach for a salt shaker. And you will avoid the effects of excess sodium in your diet such as bloating, which can lead to lethargy.

Vitamins

Vitamins are organic food substances that the body cannot manufacture. They contribute to the biochemical reactions that convert food into energy and assist in forming bone and tissue. Each vitamin has a specific task. It isn't necessary to define each one at this time; however, the important thing to remember is that if you're deficient in all or part of a single vitamin, your body's biochemical reactions may be changed causing you some major problems.

The best sources for vitamins are fresh green and yellow vegetables, fresh fruits, whole grains, fish, poultry, and meat. To ensure that you're getting all of the vitamins you need, I strongly suggest that you consider taking a daily multivitamin.

Minerals

Found in a wide range of plant and animal foods and in fresh drinking water, minerals are organic elements in their simplest form. As with vitamins, if you lack just one mineral, your body will not function properly. Minerals combine with vitamins to form enzymes that are necessary to nearly every physiological process, as well as all body tissues and internal fluids. In short, you need minerals for your body to function at peak performance. That's why you hear, "Take your vitamins and minerals every day." Minerals are not secondary supplements. They are essential elements for maintaining a healthy, active body.

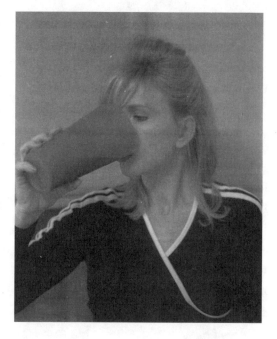

Water

Water makes up nearly 60 percent of your total body weight and is essential for:

- proper digestion
- proper absorption
- proper circulation
- proper elimination
- transportation of nutrients

* maintenance of body temperature
* maintenance of the electrolyte balance your body needs for survival
* the healthy functioning of every living cell

Vigorous physical activity causes heavy sweating—the loss of body fluid/water. Evaporation of sweat on the skin is the body's natural, built-in cooling system. However, with this loss of water comes a loss of electrolytes—ionized salts in the blood, tissue fluids and cells, including sodium, potassium, and chlorine. The depletion of these elements can cause metabolic and/or neurological difficulties.

Therefore, it is vitally important that you drink plenty of water! Most experts recommend six to eight glasses per day. During hard training, I suggest that you drink even more water. Have a glass next to you all day long and sip it often.

No nutrient acts alone. They must all be present for your body to function well at peak performance. How much is enough for you? That depends on your age, sex, size, and activity level. Good nutrition means providing your body with proper nutrients in proper amounts so that you can go about the task of daily performance.

Balancing It Out

The body works best when you feed it the right combination of food. The question is, how do you do that? The answer is by eating a variety of food from each of the four major food groups: meats, fish, and poultry; fruits and vegetables; grains, nuts and cereal; and dairy products—and by determining what percentage of your total caloric intake must come from proteins, carbohydrates, and fat sources. It is impossible for anyone to give you an exact ratio of carbohydrates, proteins, and fats because we are all created just a little bit differently. It is up to you to experiment and discover these ratios for yourself.

To find your nutritional requirements, I recommend that you keep a food journal in which you can record your daily intake of food. In your journal you might include how you feel after eating each food. Do you feel energized or do you feel like you need a nap? Do you feel bloated or lean? This information will help you discover what food your body really needs.

Calories

A calorie is a measurement of the amount of energy contained in food. Proteins and carbohydrates contain approximately four calories per gram; fats contain nine calories per gram. Though fats are the most efficient fuel when it comes to caloric density, they are the most undesirable if you are on a low-calorie program for weight control or weight reduction. If you take in more calories than your body can burn off, the excess is stored in the form of fat (adipose cells) distributed throughout the body.

It doesn't matter whether the excess is in the form of proteins, carbohydrates, or fats, your body will break it down and store it for a future time when it requires more energy than your food intake at that time is providing. Then, your body will retrieve and metabolize the fat in the adipose cells to make up the difference. If your body has all of the nutrients it needs to function optimally and if you are eating at least the minimum quantity of the various foods required at any given time by your digestive and energy producing systems, fat gain and fat loss are a matter of simple arithmetic. Unfortunately, most diets do not take these factors into consideration and that can cause a number of undesirable things to happen:

* Your body can begin to metabolize muscle tissue
* Your body's ability to metabolize fat may be impaired
* You may realize various vitamin and mineral deficiencies
* You may experience a lack of energy
* You may even develop some psychological problems

Because of the possibility of these problems, any diet regime (whether for weight gain or loss) has to take into account the body's need for certain nutritional minimums and for a relative balance of various foods in the daily food intake. The diet must be balanced in order to cause a positive reaction. Balance is the key.

So, how important are calories? Food energy comes from carbohydrates, proteins, and fats. Calories are a way of measuring the energy these nutrients provide, and there are two main points to consider in reference to calories:

* The maintenance of an ideal body weight
* Supplying an adequate amount of energy

Defining calories is really quite simple. The food you eat is converted into glycogen, and then stored in the muscles for fuel to be burned when you need it. Any excess calories are stored in the body as fat. The main question about calories is, "How many calories should I consume?" Again, that depends on individual factors such as age, gender, height, weight, activity level, and individual metabolism. These varying conditions are precisely why it is impossible for one diet plan to work for everybody. These factors are different for each of us and that is why I stress the importance of individualism when developing a nutrition program.

Since most of the people I consult are concerned with losing body fat, I have seen a host of unhealthy starvation methods, and it concerns me. Starving only creates more problems. It causes your body to feed on its own muscle, causing you to lose muscle mass. Starvation also causes your metabolism to slow down, making it even more difficult to burn fat. A good healthy nutrition program allows you to eat healthy foods in comfortable amounts for your body. In order to lose body fat, you need to feed your body steadily. Don't starve it. By feeding your body carefully and steadily, you will increase your metabolic rate, increase your body's ability to burn fat, and repair and build muscle.

To get a handle on how many calories your body burns, experiment with your calorie consumption and you will be on your way to mastering weight control. Even when you are inactive, your body still requires energy to repair and maintain cells, build muscle, and carry on basic functions, such as breathing and digestion. Therefore, it is crucial that you consume enough of the right kinds of calories to keep your body in top working order.

Calories are important to your training program in that too many calories can cause your body to retain fat; too few calories cause you to lose energy. And eating too much of a good thing can be bad as well. I have heard people say, "Eat all of the healthy food you want," or "I can have all of the fruit I want." Then, they set out to prove it by eating a whole watermelon or a serving bowl of fruit. You can gain weight if you eat too much of any food. Overload your body with anything from lettuce to chocolate bars and your body will be forced to store the excess as fat. It's just that simple.

Eating And Training

Resistance training combined with cardiovascular training puts specific nutritional demands on the body. The amount of calories you burn when training depends on your individual statistics (height, weight, etc.), the kind of activity you're doing, the intensity level of the activity, and the frequency of training sessions. The important points to remember when selecting your foods are:

* Eat a variety of foods from each of the four major food groups: meats, fish, poultry; fruits and vegetables; grains; and dairy products
* Eat the proper proportions of proteins, carbohydrates, and fats for your body.

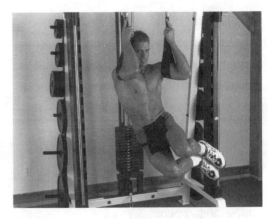

Meals

When you eat is as important as what you eat. When setting up your eating program, give strong consideration to the following criteria: your training level, your lifestyle, and your goals. The keys to remember when structuring your eating plan is to spread your meals out over the course of the day and don't skip them.

Pretraining Meals

The foods you consume before training will play a major part in how well you train. Pretraining meals help provide energy for your muscles and stock your system with fluids. They should consist of fruits, cooked vegetables, lean meats, and whole wheat breads. Pretraining meals are best eaten 1 1/2 to 2 hours before training. Pay careful attention to portions. Overeating causes loss of energy and bloating.

It's important to remember that what you eat each and every day affects your performance, not just the pretraining meals. If you don't eat a good diet consistently, your body will not be able to perform at optimal levels.

Getting Started

Your main nutritional concern should be to achieve a clean, balanced diet. This doesn't mean "going on a diet" in the old sense. Old-fashioned diets don't work. They rob your body of valuable nutrients, and they cause you to get fat.

Your body is a survival machine. Deprive it of nutrients and food, and it will find a way to survive. The body compensates for starvation by clinging to existing body fat, adding new body fat by slowing the metabolism, and inhibiting the body's natural body fat-burning process.

Nutrition doesn't have to be confusing. To become your own nutritionist, you need to get in touch with your body. You don't have to be a scientist to know that you shouldn't eat every bite on your plate even after your stomach feels full. You should be able to recognize signals, such as bloating, fullness, depression, lethargy, and anxiety. These are ways that your body uses to communicate with you about the negative effects of the foods you're eating. If you feel good, satisfied, and energetic after a meal, then you've found food that is good for your body.

In order to get in touch with your body's nutritional needs, you are going to have to get an overview of your existing nutritional habits. You begin by carefully analyzing several key points about your present diet.

The most critical components of nutrition center around:

* What you eat
* When you eat
* Why you eat
* Where you eat

The answers you come up with will expose your current nutritional patterns, which may not support your desire to reach peak performance.

Pay attention to what you eat. Read labels and record what you eat in your journal.

By tracking when you eat, you may be able to identify negative eating patterns, such as late night snacking. Do you eat most of your foods late in the day?

Why you are eating is probably the most important nutritional factor because it will tell you the real reason your body is in the shape it is now. Before you eat, ask yourself questions such as, "Am I really hungry?" Or "Am I just bored or lonely?" Or "Am I eating because my body needs fuel or energy?"

Where you eat refers to the actual location. Are you eating at fast food hamburger stands? School? Home?

These important journal entries will expose many of

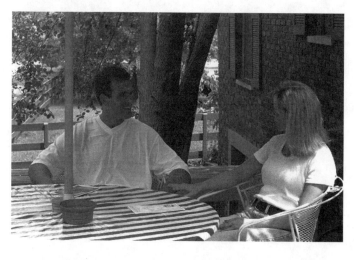

your nutritional problems—areas that need to be changed. But you won't have to change everything at once. This only causes unnecessary stress.

For starters just become aware of your nutritional habits. Eat at least three meals a day. And never skip breakfast.

Think of your body as a car. The foods you eat are the fuel. Carbohydrates and fats are like gasoline. Your body burns them for energy. Protein is like a building block and is responsible for building muscles. Vitamins and minerals derived from the foods you eat as well as supplements (which I discuss in the chapter) are like the wax on a car. They protect you from the elements. In cars this translates into rust and corrosion. For the body, this is illness and fatigue.

Chapter 7
The Importance Of Supplements

As the saying goes, an apple a day keeps the doctor away. The problem is that the apple might not be what you think it is. It could have preservatives or have been treated with pesticides or grown in nutrient-poor soil. Even when you do your best to eat a balanced diet, factors beyond your control can affect the food you eat. That is why I recommend dietary supplements.

Supplements are the safest, most effective way to ensure that your body is getting all the vital nutrients it needs to perform at its best. Today, there are a variety of supplements on the market available in nutrition stores, health food stores, and by mail order.

Are Supplements "Miracle Workers"?

Though manufacturers would like for you to believe so, supplements are not miracle or wonder products. They are merely concentrated food sources—protein, carbohydrates, fats, minerals, and vitamins.

Nutritional supplementation can be very complicated

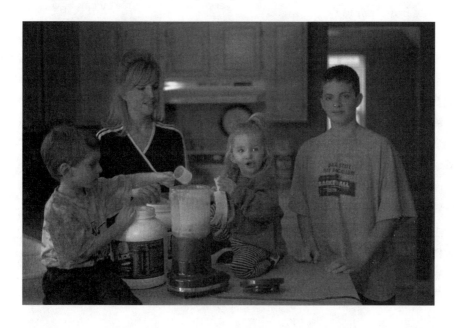

and confusing. I am constantly sorting through all the hype and testing new products. And the debate over the real benefits of supplementation continues. The pro-supplement group is typically made up of athletes and top trainers who claim that there are benefits to supplementing your diet. The anti-supplement group is typically made up of people who are not athletes, including some doctors, nutritionists, and dietitians who say that if you eat right, you won't need to supplement your diet. Round and round they go creating confusion.

When I use supplements, I feel better. My body is leaner. I'm stronger and I recover from my training sessions more quickly. Therefore, I continue to use them and recommend them to all my clients.

Supplements are important because they:

* Ensure that your body gets an adequate supply of nutrients which are essential for energy, growth, repair, and recovery
* Help your body to recover more quickly from training
* Help to control cravings and wean you from undesirable foods

Choosing Supplements

Today's supplements are far improved over the ones that were available when I was younger. The products now available mix easily, taste like a really good milkshake, and are widely available. Supplement manufacturers offer a wide variety of flavors, packaging, and mixing options as well. Their products have advanced way beyond simple protein powders.

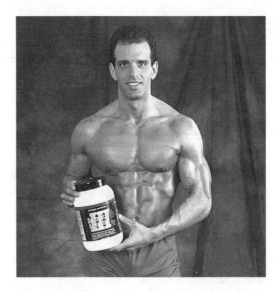

Yet with all the manufacturers stating that their products are the best and with new products coming out almost daily, choosing supplements can be very confusing. When choosing supplements, individual considerations should be taken into account, such as personal characteristics, body type, individual needs, and training goals. Choosing supplements wisely in most cases means getting help from the experts, but not everyone can give expert advice. I have found that if you stick with the products manufactured by the top companies, you really can't go wrong.

Before you go into a store, get your goals in mind and read the product labels. Most are self-explanatory. And by all means ask for advice from the people who work in the stores; it's their business to know the products that they sell.

Note: Stay away from products that promise results that seem too good to be true, such as lose 30 pounds in a week or put on 20 pounds of muscle in three days. In most cases these are tricks to get you to buy low quality products (in most cases).

Guidelines For Using Supplements

Everyone should use supplements in addition to eating regular meals. I do not recommend that you use supplements as meal replacements. My clients still eat three meals a day, even though they use supplements. The supplements are used for between meal and nutritious before-bedtime snacks.

Supplements that offer good combination of nutrients—vitamins, minerals, complex carbohydrates, proteins, fats, and special ingredients for growth, repair, and recovery—are the way to go. These products are available in powder form in a wide variety of flavors. They also offer users many options for mixing, baking, and drinking.

I also like many of the nutrition bars that are currently on the market. I have found through my own use that these work well as in between meal snacks and are tasty little desserts for after meals. They're also very handy to take along when you're on the go.

Again, the rule of thumb is to stick with products from the top manufacturers.

My Favorite Way To Take Supplements

Buying vitamins, minerals, proteins, and recovery ingredients separately is very confusing and can be extremely time consuming. Scientists and manufacturers have done us a big favor by developing all inclusive supplements. They've taken the guesswork out of the complicated science of nutritional supplementation.

All inclusive formulas such as Optimum Nutrition's Opti Rx powder combine all the vitamins, minerals, proteins, fats, carbohydrates, and special recovery ingredients into an easy-to-blend shake mix.

Give my shake recipe a try by mixing the following ingredients in a blender:

> 6-8 medium ice cubes
> 6-8 ounces of skim milk
> 1-2 scoops of supplement powder (see label for recommended serving)
> 1 banana
> Blend for 60 seconds.

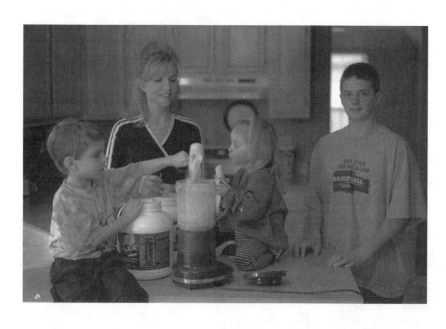

Voilà—the easiest, best-tasting way to take supplements.

Don't Break The Bank

If you have been in a nutrition store or sporting goods store that sells supplements, you were probably shocked at many of the prices. Some of these supplements are really expensive.

There is no reason to break the bank. Many of the really good supplements are not the most expensive. Optimum Nutrition's High Performance Optimizer powder comes in a 3.2 pound container and will last a couple of months. It sells for $23.95, which is very reasonable when you figure the cost per serving, and it's a lot healthier than a bag of chips.

Who Should Take Supplements

✸ Those who want to be healthy, control weight, safely lose weight, gain weight, exercise, and eat right

✸ Those involved in sports, training, and intensive exercise

✸ Those who want to ensure that the body is getting all the nutrients it needs to grow, perform, repair itself, and recover from the stresses of exercise, activity, and every day living

Chapter 8
Secrets Of Training Longevity

Many clients have asked me how I have managed to stay in top physical condition for the past 15 years. I am happy to share my secret, but the simplicity of it causes many to doubt. People assume I work out many hours everyday, but that is far from the truth. We have over-complicated diet and exercise and health. What is the secret of training longevity? One word: cycles.

I know what you're thinking, "Cycles? What does he mean by that? Is he nuts?" Let me explain.

When I was in retail exercise equipment sales, we had periods that were more sales oriented. Summers were not very busy times. From November to March was work, work, work. We sold 80% of our yearly sales during that time. Then in the spring sales would taper off. There was a season for selling—a cycle. If I were starting a business and I kept selling more and more and I kept pushing and pushing, pretty soon I'd be a burnt-out salesman. There's no back-up, no recovery time, no ease time.

Many, many people, and you may have been one of them, start exercise programs with great enthusiasm. Believing more is better, they work and work. Then after a few months, they crash. They're burnt out. They stop exercising altogether. They weren't working in cycles.

Frank Zane, the best example of cyclical training I have ever seen, explains in his book *Fabulously Fit Forever*. "Winter," says Zane, "is the period of conservation, hibernation, and inactivity. Spring is the time of rebirth, renewal, awakening and new growth. Summer is the time of warmth, light, energy, and activity. Fall is the time for maturity, harvest, and thanksgiving." Years ago when I wanted to get in shape, I went to him to learn. One of the things he taught me was you have to train in cycles. You can't carry a peak all the time. In the winter he would train less because his energy wasn't as high and the days weren't as long. In the spring he would be rejuvenated because of the sunlight and the warmth, so he would start to pick his training up. In the summer, he felt great, the days were long, he had a lot of energy and he would train a lot. In the fall he would taper back and let everything mature for the year.

He's followed that cycle for over 25 years now, so I started to implement that, too. I found it was truly the secret to training longevity. Your body gets periods of rest, and is less prone to injuries. It is also refreshing for your mind, you are less likely to become bored because you're not always doing the same thing. Psychologically, it really energizes your motivation by backing off. In other words, sometimes you're going to go back a step to go forward three steps.

All training cycles, however, do not have to follow the seasons. Sometimes schedules don't allow for seasonal cycles. When I'm on the road, I've found many small cycles are effective. I pick 4 to 6 weeks to train lighter, then 4 to six weeks to step up the training. You're always changing the cycle. Learning to make those adjustments, to follow the wave of a cycle, is the key.

If your training becomes too rigid, it will break. That is true not only of training, but also of life. Training is part of life and when training interferes with life, that means conflict. That means problems. If you can learn to take your training and adapt it to ride the wave of life, then you've just learned the secret.

Chapter 9
Stretching And Flexibility

Stretching is one of the easiest ways to improve posture, relieve tightness and tension, and add shape to the body.

Stretching exercises are without a doubt the easiest exercises to execute in any training program. They're easy to do, require little effort, and you don't need equipment or fancy facilities. And they even can be done at any level of skill.

Stretching can be defined as the act of extending beyond the current limits. Stretching results in flexibility. Flexibility can be defined, for our purposes, as the range of motion of a joint or limb. Stretching the muscles of the body allows the joints to become more pliable. Then the limb moves more freely, and the range of motion increases.

Stretching is not only good for improving the range of motion of the joints, but stretching has many other benefits including:

* Improving strength through the range of motion
* Preventing muscle soreness and injuries
* Helping shape and define muscles
* Relieving tension

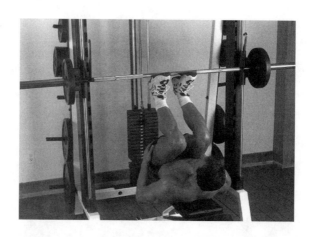

Stretching And Training

Stretching and training go hand-in-hand. Flexibility greatly improves one's ability to perform movement. Tight, rigid, inflexible muscles and joints cause one to perform sluggishly, inhibit technique, and dull the skills, which often results in aches, soreness, pain, and injuries. One of the best ways to improve your training is by stretching. Stretching is also an important ingredient of developing strong, powerful, shapely, defined and well-toned muscles.

Stretching before training helps prepare the joints and muscles for motion and helps avoid needless injuries. Stretching during training, helps keep the target area warm and limber, and it also creates awareness or that "pump feel" in the muscle or muscles being trained. Stretching after training is a great way to cool down from training and prevent muscle soreness.

My Rules For Safe And Effective Stretching
- Stretch before, during, and after training
- Never bounce, jerk, or bob...ease slowly into each stretch
- Hold each stretch for 15-30 seconds
- Always stretch the entire body during every training session
- Avoid stretches that cause pain beyond temporary discomfort
- Increase the range of motion in each new training session
- Stretch extra-tight areas twice

The following stretches have become my favorites over the years. Keep in mind, there are many stretching exercises. However, I have discovered that these work well for my clients and me. Give them a try, and if you like them, add them to your program.

Neck Stretch (Repeat opposite side)

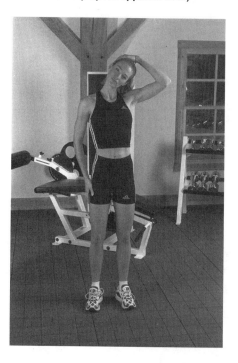

Chest Stretch

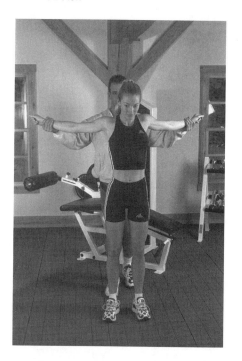

Two-Arm Pull Lat Stretch

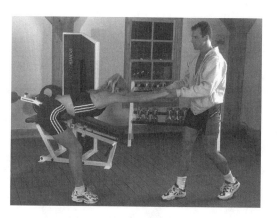

Face Down/Arms Up Shoulder Stretch

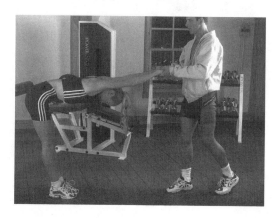

One-Arm Overhead/Tricep Stretch (Repeat Opposite Side)

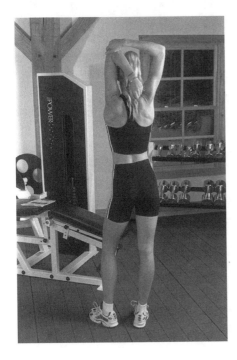

Two-Arm Back/Bicep Stretch

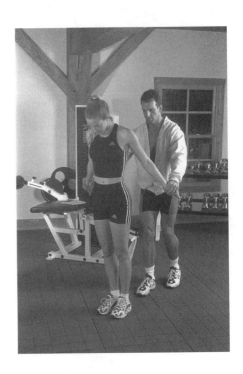

Lower Back and Hamstring Stretch

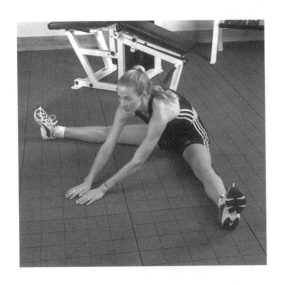

Leg Forward Hamstring Stretch (Repeat Opposite Side)

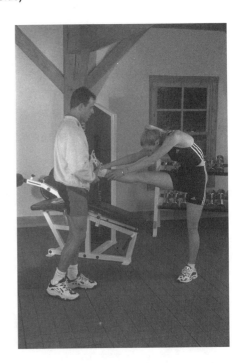

One-Leg Up/Quadricep Stretch (Repeat Opposite Side) **Calf Stretch (Repeat Opposite Side)**

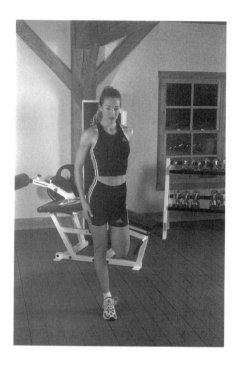 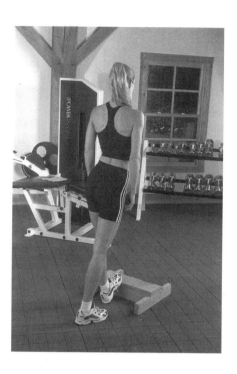

Conclusion

You will only get out of stretching what you put into it. Take it seriously. Apply the guidelines that I gave you: Always stretch before, during, and after training, and you will enjoy the many benefits of good flexibility.

Chapter 10
Beginning Weight Training Program

For weight training to be effective, you must perform the exercises properly. The best way to learn proper execution is by starting with the basics. You should think of your initial attempts at weight training as a discovery phase. It's a time when you'll discover a great many things about your body, as well as what exercises work for you and those that don't.

It's important to remember when weight training that more is not always better. Our goal in weight training is not to build huge muscles so that you can kick sand in somebody's face. The goals of the sound weight training program should include:

* Build a solid foundation of strength, muscle mass, power, muscle tone, symmetry, and endurance.
* Learn the basics of weight training exercise, techniques, and routines.
* Rehabilitate injured, lagging, or weak muscles.

There are literally thousands of weight training exercises. However, I have my favorite exercises that I use with beginners.

There are two classifications of weight training exercises—basic and isolation.

Basic exercises stress the largest muscle groups of the body—thighs, back, and chest—often in combination with smaller muscles. My favorite movements include the bench press, lat pulldowns, shoulder presses, and leg presses.

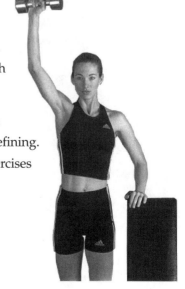

Isolation exercises stress a single muscle group or part of a single muscle. These exercises are good for shaping and defining. Leg extensions and leg curls are examples of two great exercises for shaping and defining the thighs.

Beginner Weight Training Exercises
The following are basic exercises that work well for the beginning stages of training.

Chest Press

The basic exercise for the chest is the bench press, sometimes called the chest press. This is sometimes called the king of the upper body exercises because it is one of the best. It primarily stresses the chest muscles with a secondary emphasis on the front of the shoulders and the back of the arms. You can perform this exercise on the chest press machine (shown below), or by using barbells, dumbbells, or a Smith Machine.

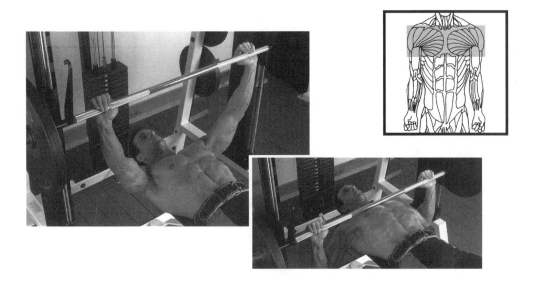

Lat Machine Pulldown

The most basic exercise for the back is the lat machine pulldown. This exercise places direct stress on the upper muscle of the back and is famous for helping develop the V-shape look of the body. The lat pulldown also helps tone and shape the biceps and forearm muscles.

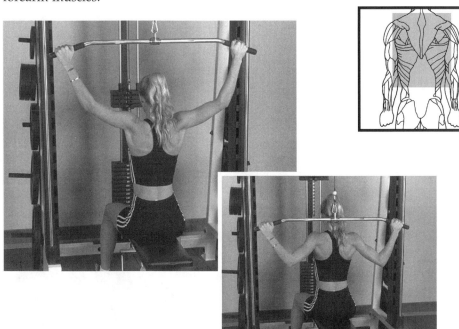

Shoulder Press

The granddaddy of the shoulder exercises, the shoulder press involves pressing a weight overhead, stressing the entire shoulder girdle and putting secondary stress on the triceps.

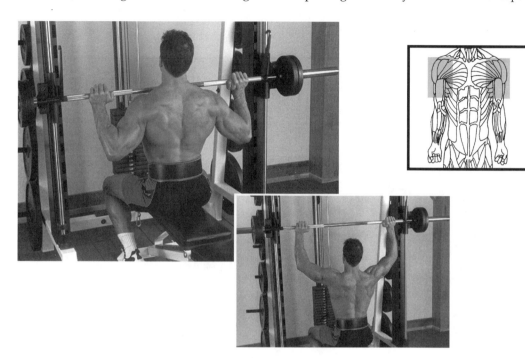

Arm Curl

The arm curl is the most basic exercise for the biceps. It involves curling a barbell or dumbbell in a semicircular arc to a position just beneath the chin, then lowering it to the starting point in front of the hips.

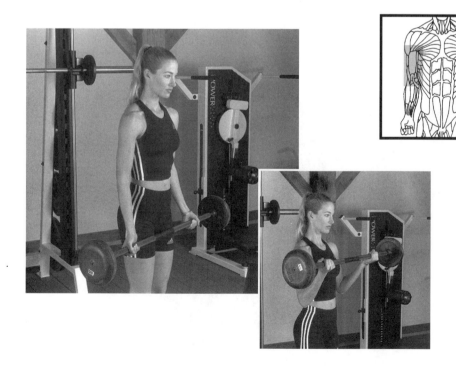

Tricep Extension

This is the most basic exercise for the triceps, although tricep press movements are also good.

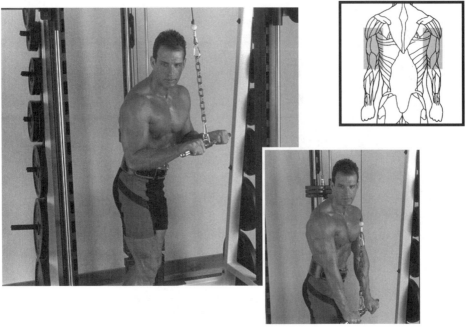

Leg Press

While the squat is by far the best exercise for the legs, it takes a great deal of control and balance that can only be acquired with experience. Therefore, I start beginners out on the leg press.

The leg press is performed on a machine. Very much like the squat, the leg press stresses the entire leg region without putting much pressure on the lower back. You do not have to balance the weight; therefore, it is safer to perform and allows you to build good foundation of strength which will enable you to perform squats as you advance in your program.

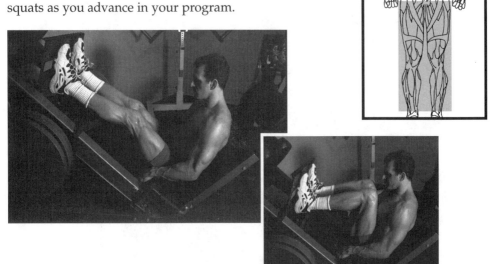

Leg Extension

The leg extension is an isolation exercise that puts a strong emphasis on the upper thigh muscles — the quadriceps. Although it is not labeled as a basic exercise, I find it's helpful in the beginning stages of training.

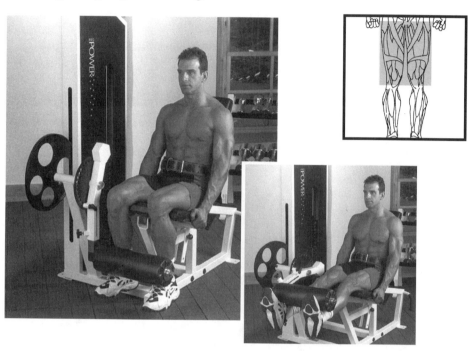

Leg Curl

The leg curl is also labeled an isolation exercise. It is the counterpart to the leg extension affecting the upper rear or hamstring area.

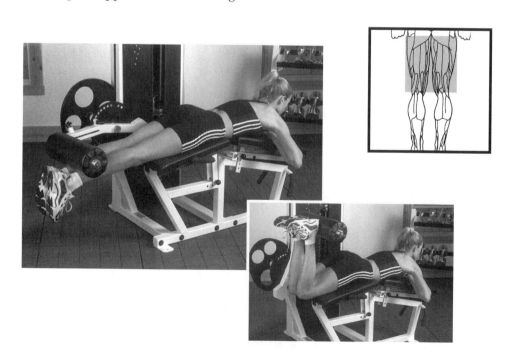

Standing Calf Raise

Calf exercises are often left out of many weight training programs, but they shouldn't be. In women, the underdevelopment of the calf can cause the thigh and hips to appear large and pear shaped.

For men, the calves are just as important, especially for defining the classic physique. Measurements of the neck, calves, and biceps are used to help determine the symmetry of the body. For sports, the calves are important in running, jogging, sprinting, and jumping.

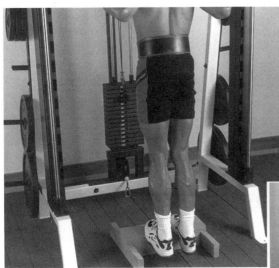
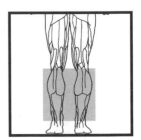
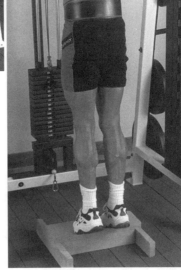

Four-Way Neck Isometrics

This is an isolation exercise that you can use to strengthen the neck muscles. It's an easy, safe way to strengthen the neck muscles and does not require any equipment.

Many people have underdeveloped or weak necks. This can prevent you from properly performing shoulder presses, squats, and stomach crunches. Therefore, it's important to develop your neck muscles if they are weak.

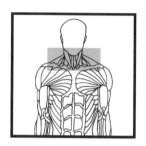

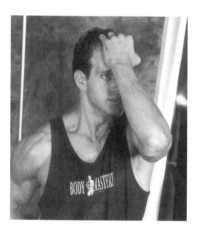
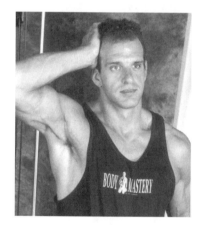
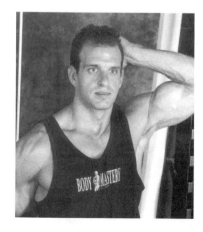
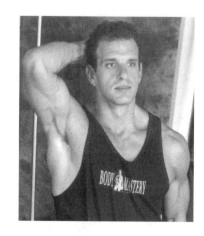

Partial Incline Sit-Up

I haven't met anyone yet who is not concerned with the midsection or waist. The partial incline sit-up uses only the upper 65 percent range of the sit-up movement. When performed correctly, this exercise stresses the upper and lower abdominals with no pressure on the lower back.

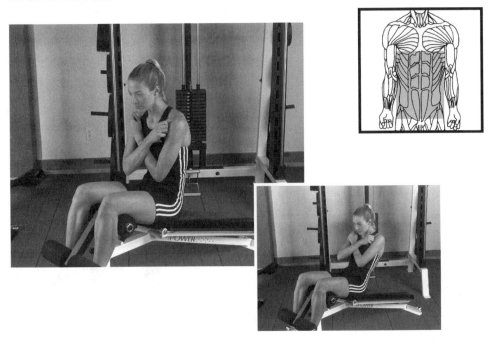

Hyperextensions

Lower back training is always essential at any level. It is extremely important in the beginning stages of training because a weak lower back will eventually become a big problem. The hyperextension is excellent for strengthening the lower back region. It is easy and safe and requires no equipment, so it can be performed anywhere.

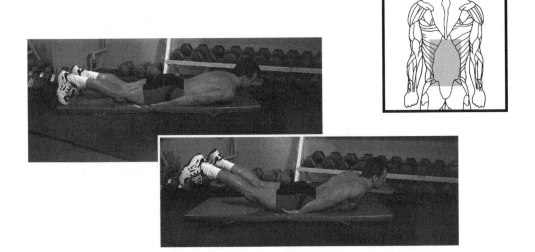

Starting Out

Beginners should train for technique, muscle coordination, and endurance. This is accomplished by performing 10 to 25 repetitions of each exercise. It is not a good idea to train for muscle strength, power, and mass as a beginner. After you gain experience, develop balance, and good weight lifting form, you can begin experimenting with heavier weights.

First things first—keep your focus on familiarizing yourself with these basic exercises and pay attention on how your body is responding to the training.

Weight Training Techniques

Weight training techniques are the specific ways in which you perform weight training movements. At the beginner level, I have five favorites.

Same Weight Straight Sets

This is a good technique to use while learning the groove or movement of each lift. To perform this technique, use a moderate amount of weight and perform the lifting exercise for three sets, with ten to fifteen reps per set. The weight remains the same for each set. After completing three sets, move onto the next exercise. This technique is excellent for teaching form because by lifting the same amount of weight throughout the three sets, you are able to concentrate more on technique than on how much weight you are lifting.

Example:

1 set 10-15 reps with 100 pounds
1 set 10-15 reps with 100 pounds
1 set 10-15 reps with 100 pounds

Isolation Sets

This technique works a muscle or muscle group completely before moving onto another muscle or muscle group.

Example:

Perform one set of eight reps on the leg press machine.
Rest thirty seconds.
Perform a second set.
Rest thirty seconds.
Perform a third set, and then move onto a new exercise.

Progressive Overload

This is really the goal behind weight training. Making your muscles work harder is the basis behind building strength, toning muscles, and increasing muscular endurance. In performing this technique, you overload the muscles by steadily increasing the poundage, and/or by adding sets and reps throughout the sequence of lifts. You may also perform this technique by increasing the frequency of weight training sessions, changing exercises, or using a variety of techniques.

Circuit Training

This is very popular with beginners. When you perform a series of weight training exercises in a circuited manner—one after another—with little rest in between reps and sets, you are engaged in circuit training. Here you will go through a series of weight machines, working each body part for one set, then repeating the circuit for another set or sets. This training technique also produces cardiovascular benefit and develops muscle endurance. It's popular because it saves time.

Priority (Weak Muscle) Training

Sometimes you must strengthen one muscle before you can train other muscles. For example, many people have weak neck muscles that won't allow them to do abdominal work. In order to work up to doing enough stomach crunches to work the abs, these people must first strengthen their neck muscles by giving the weak or lagging muscle special attention.

For instance in the case of a weak neck, I suggest adding several sets of 4-way isometrics at the end of each training session. Another example is that I have a weak rear deltoid muscle (back side of my shoulder) which is not as developed as the rest of my shoulder muscles (front and middle deltoids); therefore, I train my lagging muscle first when my attention and energy level are high. Some people center their entire workout around developing an underdeveloped or weak muscle or muscle group.

Beginning Weight Training Routines

Your training routine is the complete program you do during a single training session, including all of the aerobic training and weight training exercises.

At the beginning stages, I recommend that you train two to three times per week with a day or two of rest between each workout. Your lifestyle and goals will be factors in determining the routine you select. Your routine should be comfortable and fit easily into your lifestyle. Setting up a routine which creates anxiety is a sure road to failure. You'll either skip workouts or quit training all together. As with any new habit, it may take some time to get used a new routine, so give your training a chance before throwing in the towel.

I usually recommend the two day a week routine or the three-day a week routine. The two-day routine can be:

Monday-Thursday
Tuesday-Friday
Wednesday-Saturday

The two-day routine work well for those who have little time to devote to training, have limited access to training facilities, or who aren't overly concerned about weight loss. This is an especially good routine for beginners. Here, the entire body is trained at each workout.

Three-day routines works better for people who want to lose body fat, get in shape more quickly, and enjoy training. Generally, you'll train a different part of the body each day. For instance:

Monday, Wednesday, Friday
Tuesday, Thursday, Saturday
Wednesday, Friday, Sunday

Workout 1 - chest, shoulders, legs, abs
Workout 2 - light legs, calves, abs, biceps, triceps
Workout 3 - back, legs, abs, calves.

Sets, Reps, Weight, Intensity

As a beginner, you should focus on doing one weight training exercise per body part during each training session. For the first few sessions, do only one set per exercise. Then, as you gain confidence and become more comfortable with the exercises, you'll want to increase the number of sets until you reach four sets per exercise.

Keep your repetitions in the 10 to 15 rep range for the chest, shoulders, back, biceps, triceps, and thighs. Twelve to 25 reps work best for the neck, abdomen, lower back, and calves.

Keep the intensity of your workouts moderate by choosing weights that allow you to perform in the desired repetition range.

Breathing And Rest Between Sets

Much has been written about the way you should breath when performing a weight lifting movement. I simply recommend that you breath naturally. However, it may be helpful to exhale during the upward part of the movement or the positive portion of the lift. During the downward or negative portion of the lift, you should inhale. Just don't hold your breath. Holding your breath cuts off oxygen to the brain and could cause you to pass out. (Not a good idea when you're holding weights in each hand.)

A way to synchronize your breathing pattern is to breathe in as you lower the weigh, then say "ooh" or "ahh" as you raise the weight. Making that funny little sound will force you to exhale and prevent you from holding your breath.

Resting between reps is very important. Specific training techniques require different rest periods between reps. For instance, training for strength, power, and mass requires all-out effort, which in turn, increases the need for rest, usually two to four minutes of rest between sets. Training for muscle tone—using a moderate amount of weight—will require between one to two minutes of rest. Training for muscular endurance will require a rest period of only 30 seconds to one minute.

Your current condition will also dictate how much rest you need between sets. As you get into better shape, the need for rest will decrease. A good rule to follow is when you start to recover your breath, begin the next set. It will help you work at your current level of conditioning. As you get into better shape, the rest period adjusts naturally because the better condition you're in, the faster you recover.

A Final Note

Learning the basics is a time to learn how to lift weights. It's not a time to see how much weight the bar can hold. Rather, you should focus on learning the exercises, executing the movements, and getting a handle on your strengths and weaknesses. It's also a time for you to learn about your body and how it responds to weight training.

Chapter 11
Intermediate Weight Training

Most clients I work with reach a point when they are ready to delve deeper into the weight training portion of their program. They have learned and applied the basics that I taught them when they were beginners, but they realize that they will have to challenge themselves more with the weights in order to progress.

After beginning a training program, it doesn't take long for one to realize that lifting weights is what really produces the most dramatic changes to the body. I want to be careful not to slight the importance of aerobic training and good nutritional practices. These are very, very important in the overall picture of health and fitness. But it is the weight training that really causes the body to become more defined, shapely, and toned.

In this chapter I will share with you my favorite intermediate weight training exercises. I will also discuss intermediate level routines, talk about training techniques, sets, reps, stretching, and good ways to complement your weight training with aerobic exercise.

This information will help you elevate your training to the next level.

How Do I Know If It's Time To Advance My Weight Training?

When a program begins to get stale—you feel unchallenged, unmotivated, and your progress seems to have stalled—it is time to make a change. Usually you can tell that your program is working by simply looking in the mirror. However, often it's more difficult to see when the body stops making progress. The lack of "good" soreness after

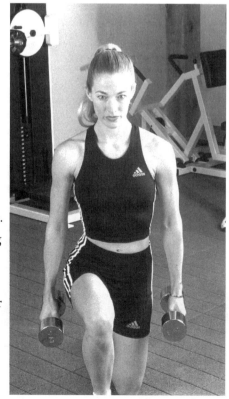

a training session is a sign that it is time to change your program.

When you first started training with weights, you probably felt sore for a couple of days after your session. As your body began getting into better shape, you began cycling through the soreness more quickly until eventually you no longer felt sore after your sessions. When this happens it's time to move on to the next level so that you can begin challenging yourself to make even greater improvements.

Intermediate Weight Training Exercises
In Chapter Ten, I outlined several good beginner weight training exercises. These basic exercises—chest press, lat pulldown, shoulder press, barbell arm curl, tricep pushdown, leg press, leg extension, leg curl, calf raise, partial incline sit-up, and back hyperextension—are still great foundation-building exercises, and they should remain part of your program even as you advance to the intermediate level. Continuing to perform and master these exercises will further develop the body and continue building a solid muscular foundation.

At this level, however, I like to add isolation exercises to the routine. They are referred to as isolation exercises because they stress one muscle group or part of a muscle group. They are excellent for putting on the finishing touches, and they work well to shape, tone, and define the targeted muscle.

Intermediate Chest Exercises
The chest press is still the best basic exercise for working the pectoral muscles. At the intermediate level, you can increase the development of your pectorals by adding pressing exercises such as the incline chest press and decline chest press. You can place emphasis on specific areas of the chest by utilizing various angles in your pressing movements. At the intermediate level, I like to add flat bench dumbbell flys. Dumbbell flys are a great exercise for developing muscle detail and creating shape.

Smith Machine Chest Press (Basic Movement)

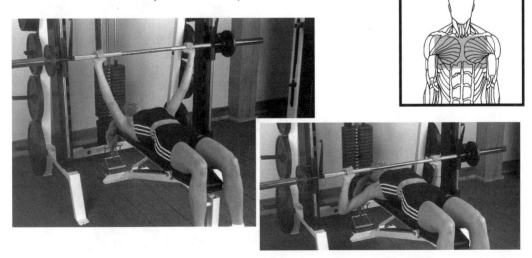

Flat Bench Dumbbell Flys (Isolation Movement)

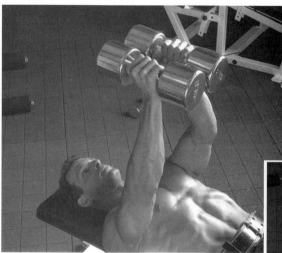
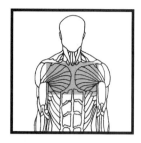
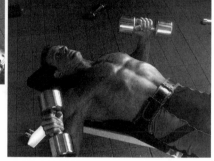

Intermediate Back Exercises

The back muscles cover a large territory and are the largest muscles in the upper body. These muscles stretch from the base of the neck to the top of the butt and go from shoulder to shoulder. In the beginning, most people find the back difficult to train because they are unable to feel the muscles when they exercise. Because the back muscles are so large and because they are usually underdeveloped, I like to stick with basic exercises in the intermediate level of training. The lat pulldown exercise should remain a staple in your program.

However, now you can add variety to the movement by changing hand grips from wide to medium to narrow, or you can change from pulling the bar to the front instead of pulling it behind the neck. There are also various attachments that you can get to change the angle and to stress different areas of the back. If your strength permits, you may incorporate chinning-type movements into your workout. Chin-ups work, but they are difficult for most people. However, if you can do them comfortably, add them to your program for variety.

Rowing is a great exercise for developing muscle thickness in the middle back and is an exercise that you can do with free weights or on a machine. Though there are many machines and exercises from which to choose, I recommend that you start this exercise on a low pulley machine.

There are many ways to work the lower back. The hyperextension, lower back weight machine, deadlifts, and partial deadlifts are all exercises that work the lower back. However, I caution you to start slowly when strengthening the lower back because it is easy to overload.

Lat Machine Pulldowns—Behind The Neck (Basic Movement)

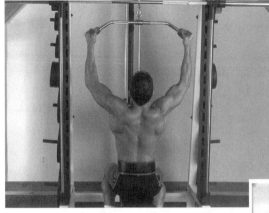
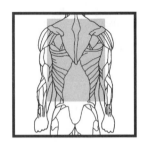
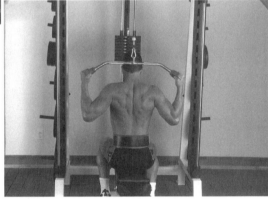

Seated Low Pulley Cable Rows (Basic Movement)

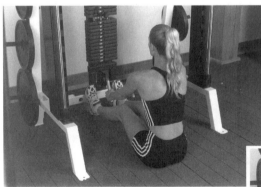
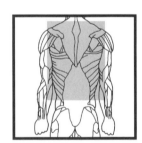
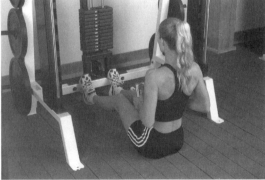

Lower Back Low Pulley Extension (Isolation Movement)

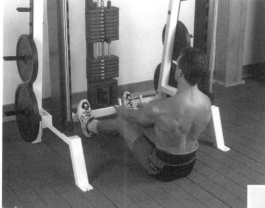
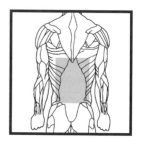
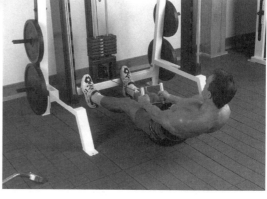

NOTE—The lower back exercise should be the last exercise you perform in your weight training session.

Intermediate Shoulder Exercises

The shoulder press should remain your primary exercise for the shoulders. However, if you want to try something different, use different pressing movements such as behind-the-neck press, dumbbell press, or machine press.

The isolation exercise for the shoulders is the lateral raise. There are three types of lateral raises—front, side, and rear. Laterals involve lifting or extending your arm in an upward arc motion.

Smith Machine Shoulder Press (Front)

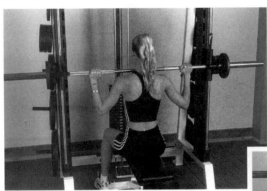
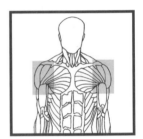
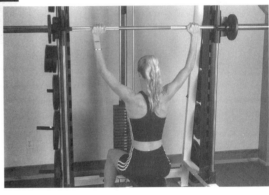

Lateral Dumbbell Raise (Isolation Movement)

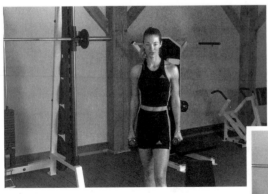
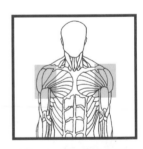
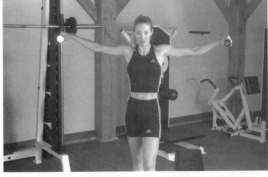

Intermediate Bicep Exercises

The best and most basic way to train the biceps is by performing bicep curls using a machine, barbell, cable, or dumbbell. Biceps also receive significant work during pulling and chinning movements.

The dumbbell arm curl is an excellent exercise for shaping and putting the finishing touches on the bicep muscle.

Barbell Arm Curl (Basic Movement)

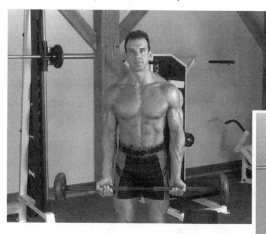
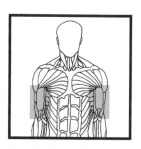
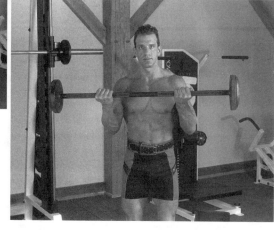

Dumbbell Arm Curl (Isolation Movement)

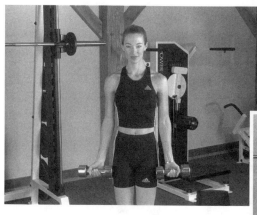
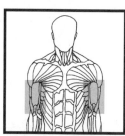
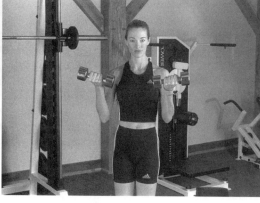

Intermediate Tricep Exercises

The tricep muscle makes up about three quarters of the arm's total size. The pushdown should remain in your program. You can vary the movement by changing hand positions or by using one of the many attachments available. This is a great exercise for overall tricep development, specifically good for increasing muscle size and strength.

Smith Machine Close Grip Press (Basic Movement)

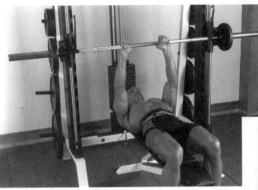
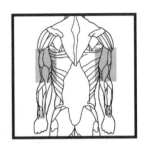
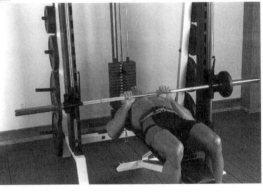

Cable Pushdowns (Isolation Movement)

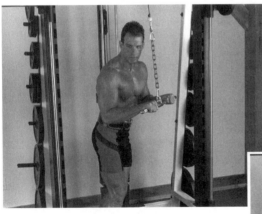
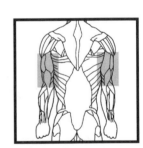
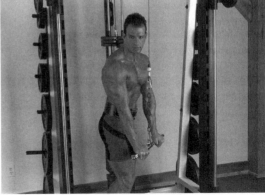

Intermediate Leg Exercises

The most basic exercise for the legs is the leg press. It is great for stressing the muscles from the waist down. The leg press emphasizes the entire lower body with specific emphasis on the quadriceps.

If you chose not to do squats as a beginner, you may want to add them to your intermediate program. If you have consistently performed leg presses in your beginner program, you have probably developed enough strength to begin squats. For the beginner, squats can be uncomfortable. They require a lot of concentration, strength, and good lung capacity. For instance, the barbell squat involves almost every major muscle of the body, making it extremely taxing. It doesn't matter whether you are a beginner or a pro, squats are always challenging.

The leg press and the squat are exercises that work well for developing strength, building mass, and toning the glutes, quadriceps, hamstrings, and calves.

The leg extension exercise is great for defining and shaping the front of the thigh, especially the knee area.

Probably the most underdeveloped muscle in the lower body region is the hamstring (back of the thigh). The best way to develop the hamstring muscle is the lying leg curl. This exercise directly emphasizes the back of the leg/hamstring muscles.

(a) Leg Press (Basic Movement)

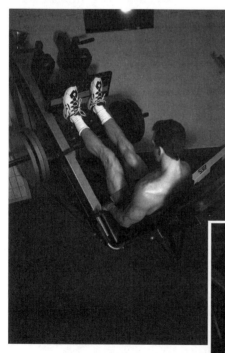

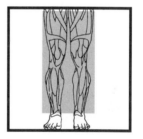

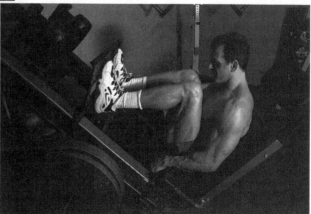

(b) Smith Machine Squat (Basic Movement)

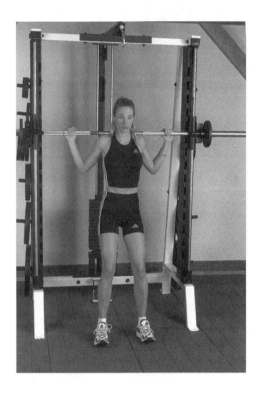
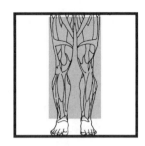
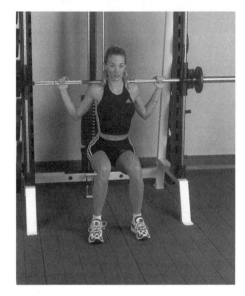

2. Leg Extensions (Isolation Movement)

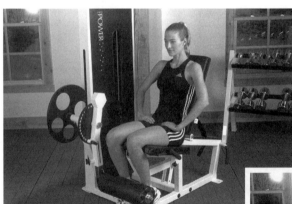
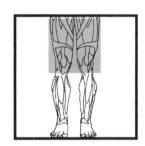
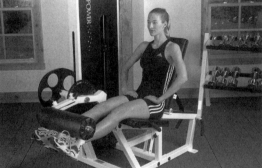

3. Leg Curls (Isolation Movement)

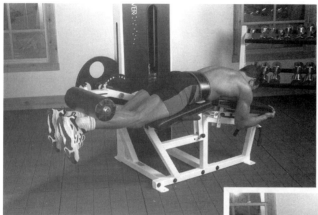
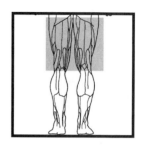

Intermediate Abdomen Exercises

It seems that everyone wants to work on their abs. The abdomen, like other areas of the body, needs special attention. The abdominals are a group of muscles that are the visual center of the body. More than any other muscle, they help define a fit body.

The abdominal muscles pull the upper body (the rib cage) and the lower body (the pelvis) toward each other, and they help to keep the internal organs in place. The rectus abdominis, a long muscle extending along the length of the abdomen, is the muscle that flexes and draws the sternum toward the pelvis. The external obliques are muscles at each side of the torso, commonly called the handles. The intercostals, two thin planes of muscular and tendon fibers that occupy the spaces between the ribs, lift the ribs and draw them together.

In training, it is common to divide the abdominals into three areas: the upper, lower, and sides.

The exercise that stresses the upper abdominal region is the crunch. The lower region of the abdominal is best exercised by performing various leg raise movements. The side muscles of the abdomen are worked best by twisting or side raises.

Exercise Suggestions:

1. Upper Abdominal—Crunches (feet on bench)

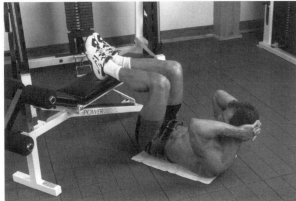
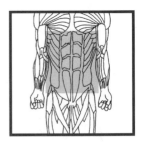
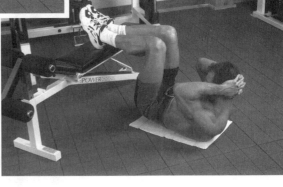

2. Lower Abdominal—Knee-ups

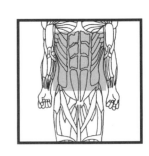
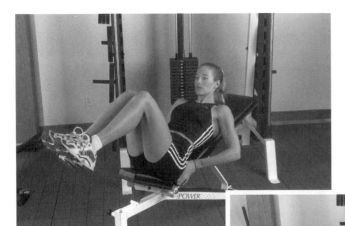

3. Sides (Obliques)—Twists

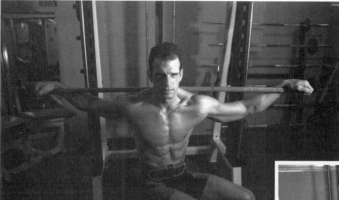
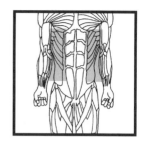
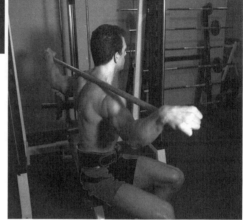

Intermediate Weight Training Techniques

There are five weight-training techniques that I like to use for intermediate training: super sets, compound sets, pyramid sets, descending sets, and reverse order sets. You can also use any of the three training techniques introduced in Chapter Ten, the beginner training program: straight sets, isolation sets, progressive overload, circuit sets, and priority training.

Super Sets

Super sets are a very popular training technique. This technique is performed by combining two exercises that work opposing muscle groups, for example, doing a set of dumbbell arm curls then doing a set of tricep pushdowns. Repeat these two exercises until you have completed the desired number of sets. You should alternate the pattern: work the bicep, work the tricep, work the bicep, work the tricep, and so forth until you have completed the proper number of sets for the workout.

Compound Sets

Compound sets are performed by rotating two exercises for the same body part, for example, do a set of barbell curls, then a set of dumbbell curls. Repeat this sequence until you have completed the desired number of sets for the workout.

Pyramid Sets

Pyramid sets enable you to train with heavy weights in a progressive, or pyramid, manner. Muscle fibers grow and get stronger by contracting against resistance. It isn't wise to just jump in and begin lifting heavy weights, but by practicing the pyramid technique you can add weight progressively as you go through the workout. For example, if 90 pounds is the ideal weight for you (ideal meaning the weight that produces the right amount of resistance to promote muscle reaction), then you would not start an exercise by lifting 90 pounds in the first set. Your muscles, joints, tendons, and ligaments wouldn't be warmed up, and you would run the risk of suffering an injury. The pyramid method allows you to start exercising at a weight lower than the maximum weight and progressively add weight until you work up to heavier weights.

Pyramid training is the best technique for developing strength/power and building muscle mass. Here's an example of pyramiding:

1 set of 12 reps with 100 pounds

1 set of 10 reps with 110 pounds

1 set of 8 reps with 120 pounds

1 set of 4 reps with 130 pounds

1 set of 2 reps with 140 pounds

This is an effective, safe way to push yourself to progress toward lifting heavier weights without running the risk of injury.

Descending Sets

The descending sets training method is accomplished by moving from lifting the heaviest weight you can lift to lowering the weight progressively for each set. This is an advanced technique that has proven very successful for those following the intermediate level program. You do need to use caution when utilizing this method and use it only once in a while.

An example of the descending set technique using the dumbbell arm curl would be to begin the first set with 35 pound weights for 10 reps, set the dumbbells in the rack, and then do the next set with 30 pounds for six reps. Then, set the 30 pound weights in the rack and do the last set with 25 pound weights for several reps until your arms are fatigued.

Reverse

Reverse order works well when your workout gets stale. This technique allows you to spruce up the workout by switching the batting order. Instead of doing your chest first and your legs last, you can switch to doing your legs first and your chest last. Instead of doing the back before doing the biceps, do the biceps first and then do the back, and so on. This technique really helps when you are feeling mentally burned out.

By incorporating the various weight training techniques into your program, you will trick your body into feeling as if it is being treated with a new program every time you work out, and that promotes positive results.

Intermediate Weight Training Routines

You will want to train a minimum of three times per week (Monday, Wednesday, Friday; or Tuesday, Thursday, Saturday; or Wednesday, Friday, Sunday). The length of the sessions will increase and you are going to feel a little more fatigued at the end of each workout than you did as a beginner.

My favorite intermediate training routine is to train chest, shoulders, triceps, and abdominals the first session; legs, calves, and abdominals the second session; and back, biceps, forearms, and abdominals on third session.

Intermediate Sets & Reps
Keep in mind, if your goal is to increase strength, select and use a weight that keeps your repetitions in the 1 to 6 range. If your goal is to tone, keep your reps in the 8 to 12 range. If you are trying to increase your muscular endurance, keep your reps in the 12 to 25 range.

Do one to three sets of each exercise with two to four minutes of rest between sets depending on your level of fitness and training goal. A good way to judge how much rest you need between sets is to perform a set, catch your breath, and then perform the next set. When you catch your breath after each set, you will know that your body is ready to start the next set. Those who are training for power/strength will want to rest for two to five minutes between each set.

Your ultimate goal should be to learn to read your body's signals well enough to know what's working in your program and what is not.

Chapter 12
Advanced Level Weight Training

Advanced training represents the pursuit of physical excellence. This level of training requires that you learn how to read your body's signals, analyze the information, and react with the right action. It means doing a lot more than just involving yourself in an exercise program.

Reacting appropriately to this feedback by altering your program accordingly until it approaches the ideal formula is the key to succeeding at the advanced level. Those who have reached this level are able to develop an instinctive feel, an internal guidance, that tells them when to train, what to train, how much to train, when to rest, when to eat, what to eat, and so forth. This often requires many hours of training and sometimes years of experimentation to learn what works best for your individual characteristics.

Moving Up To The Advanced Level
It's human nature for one to want to push the envelope, however, one should not expect to jump from an intermediate level program to an advanced level program all at once. You will need to make a slow transition from one level to the next for two reasons. First, a sudden jump in intensity may lead to injury, fatigue, and burnout. Secondly, this level of training may be more than you are ready for or want. Psychologically, it may be premature to move to this level. If so, you may stop training all together. Remember, the advanced level training program is definitely not for everyone.

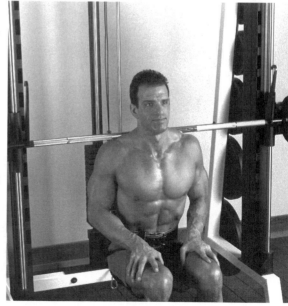

Advanced Level Training

At the advanced level, you will need to practice what Frank Zane calls intelligent training—making the most gains from the least amount of effort. The "more is better" or "no pain, no gain" approaches will only lead to imbalance, overtraining, injury, and eventual burnout. In order to avoid these problems, you will want to make your training efficient and sensible. Again, it will require that you listen to your body.

The goal for the advanced level training should be to constantly strive for a balance between muscle size, strength, definition, tone, shape, and development. In order to reach this goal, you must constantly assess your training results.

To further develop your body, you will need to master the exercises listed in Chapters 10 and 11. Also, learn and integrate into your program the new exercises introduced in this chapter.

There are so many advanced weight training exercises that I could never list all of them. However, below, I have listed the exercises that are my favorites.

Advanced Chest Exercises

To fully develop your chest, you need to pay attention to all of the areas; the inside, outside, upper, and lower areas of the pectoral. In shaping the pectoral, strive for a nice square look rather than one in which the muscle appears flat, saggy, and shapeless.

The two basic exercises for the chest are presses and flys. The chest exercises I have listed for the advanced level are designed to help you achieve complete chest development. Incorporate these exercises from each of the areas I have listed below.

Upper Chest—Incline Dumbbell Presses

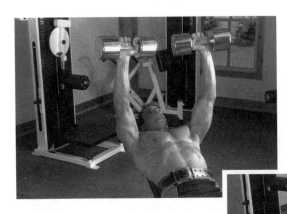
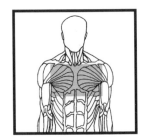

Lower Chest—Decline Barbell Presses

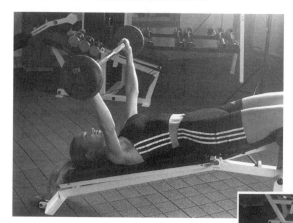
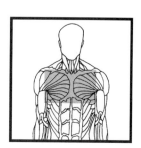

Inner Chest—Cable Crossovers

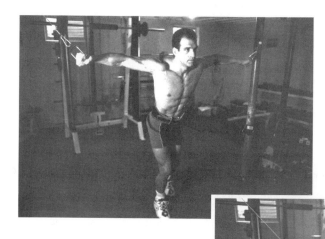
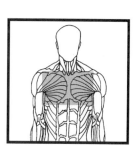

Outer Chest—Smith Machine Incline Presses (Wide Grip)

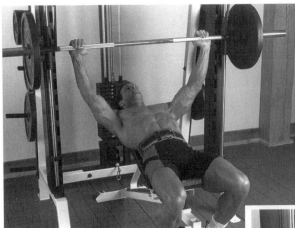
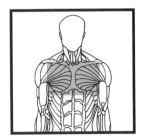
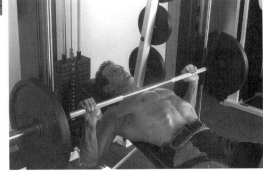

Advanced Shoulder Exercises

The deltoids enable your arm to move in a 360-degree circle, and that means that there are many angles from which to train your shoulders in order to bring out their full shape and development.

The two basic exercises for training the deltoids are presses and lateral raises. Shoulder presses begin with arms bent and the weight held about shoulder height. You then lift a barbell or dumbbells straight overhead.

Laterals involve lifting your extended arm upward in a wide arc. In order to work all three heads, you need to do laterals to the front, to the side, and to the rear. When you do laterals, you completely isolate the various heads of the deltoids. Select exercises from the key areas listed on the next pages:

Entire Shoulder Region—Barbell Shoulder Press

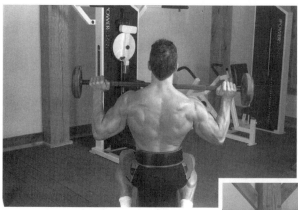
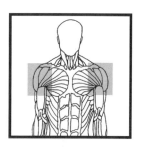
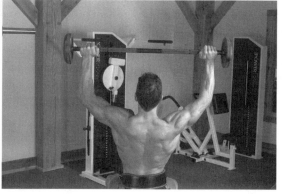

Front Deltoids (Anterior)—Dumbbell Front Raise

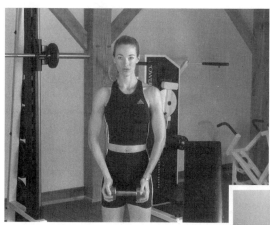
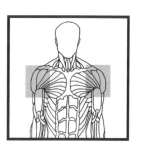

2. Middle Deltoids (Medial)—Dumbbell Incline Lateral Raise

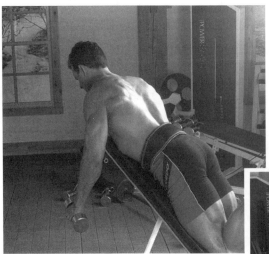
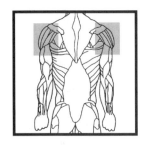
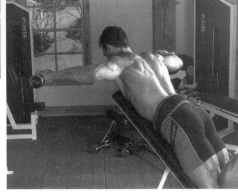

3. Rear Deltoids (Posterior)—Bent-over Lateral Raises

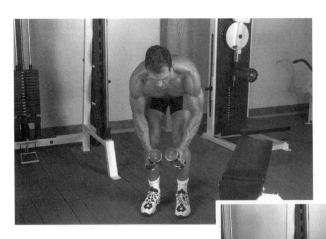
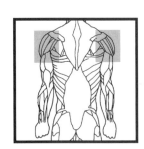

Advanced Bicep Exercises

People who relate bulging biceps with being totally in shape are wrong. Bicep size and mass are important for defining a well developed bicep muscle; however, shape, definition, and complete development are more important than pure size. Using a variety of movements to develop the complete quality of the muscle and varying your training techniques will help you achieve greater results. Choose exercises that work each of the key areas:

1. Mass Of Biceps—Standing Dumbbell Curls

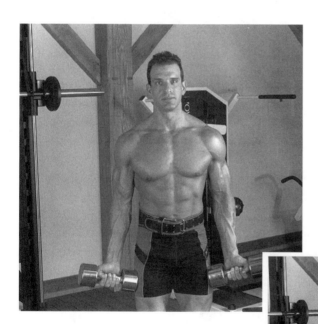

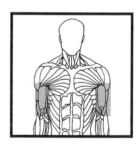

2. Length And Lower Thickness Of Biceps—Incline Dumbbell Curls

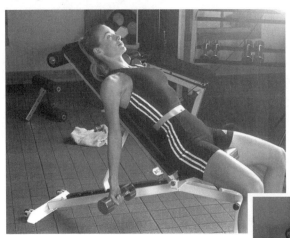
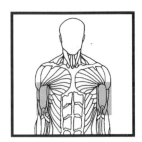

3. Height Of Biceps—Dumbbell Concentration Curls

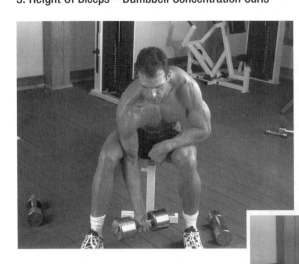
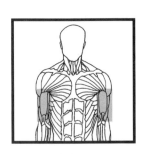

4. Outside Bicep—Reverse Barbell Curls

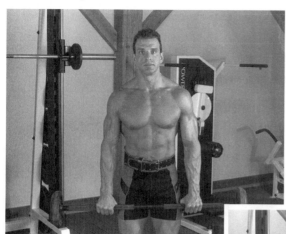
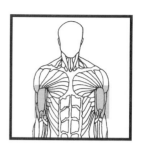

5. Inner Bicep—Standing Alternate Dumbbell Curls

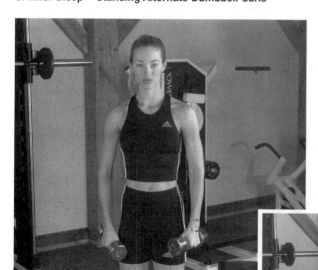
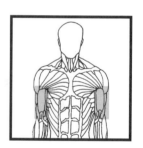

Advanced Tricep Exercises

The two ways to work the tricep muscles are pressing movements and extension movements. Even though the triceps are involved in a wide range of exercises, it is necessary—especially as you become more advanced—to isolate and stress them individually to make certain you get full development of the muscle structure. Choose exercises that work each of the key areas:

Triceps Mass—Bench Dips

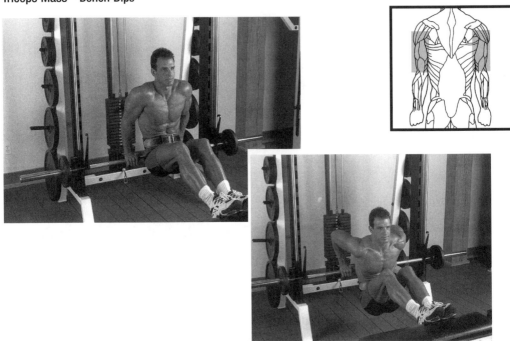

Upper Triceps—Smith Machine Overhead Extension

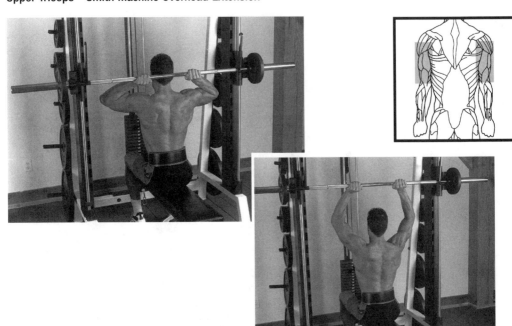

Lower Triceps—Reverse Cable Pushdown

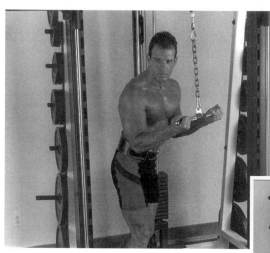
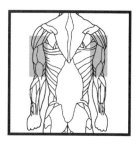
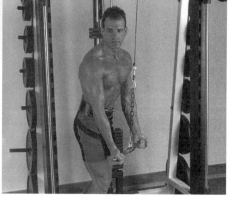

Inner Triceps—Close Grip Dumbbell Press

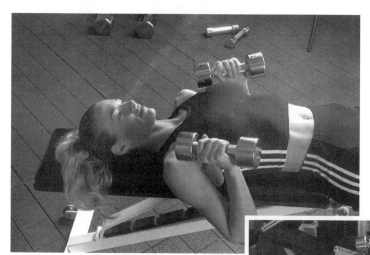
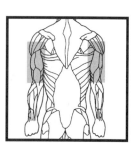

Advanced Forearm Exercises

Though often overlooked, you should consider your forearms just as important as any other body part. They are involved in nearly every upper body exercise either by helping you grip a piece of equipment or by being a part of the pushing and pulling portion of the exercise. Every time you flex the elbows or wrists, you put stress on your forearm muscles. Forearm development is important for both appearance and strength. Choose exercises that work the key areas:

Upper Forearms—Reverse Barbell Wrist Curls

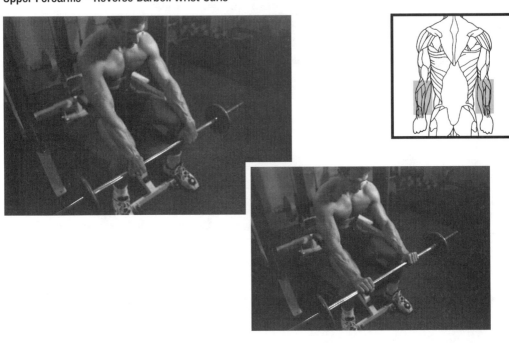

Inner Forearms—Barbell Wrist Curls

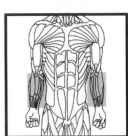

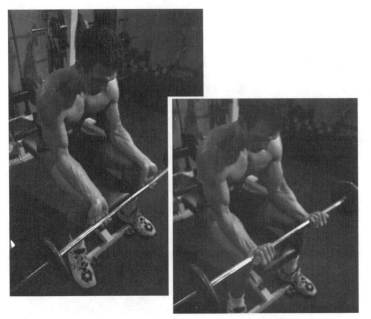

Advanced Quadricep Exercises

The best way to train the quadriceps is to divide the muscle group into three areas—lower, outer and inner—and do specific exercises that directly stress these areas individually. Choose exercises that work each of the key areas:

Lower Quadriceps—Leg Extensions

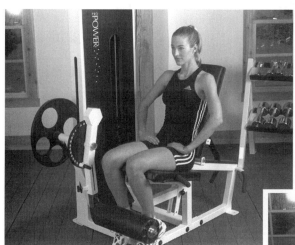
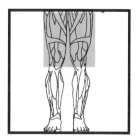
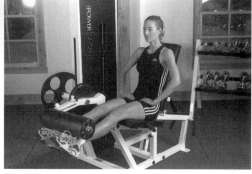

Outer Quadriceps—Machine Hack Squats (feet pointed straight ahead, close together)

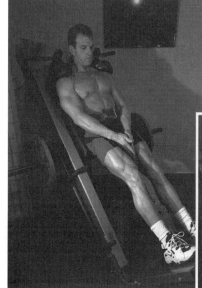
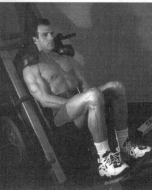
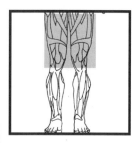

Inside Quadriceps—Smith Machine Squat (feet relatively wide apart, toes pointed out)

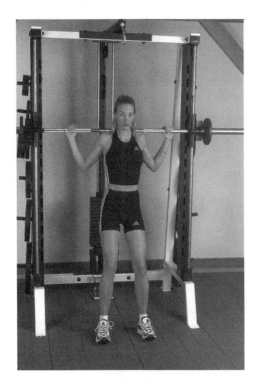
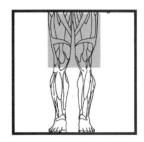
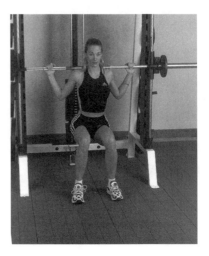

Advanced Hamstring Exercises

An advanced exercise that works well for developing the hamstring:

Dumbbell stiff leg deadlift

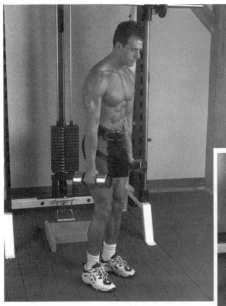
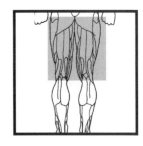
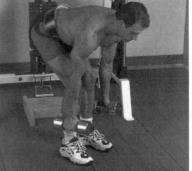

Advanced Buttock Exercises

The primary muscles of the buttocks are the gluteus maximus and the gluteus medius. The gluteus maximus contracts to help straighten the legs and torso from a completely or partially flexed position.

Smith Machine Lunges

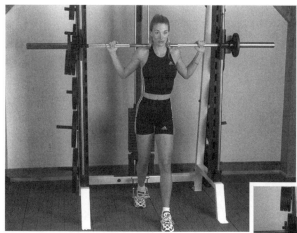
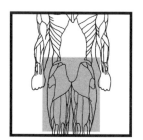
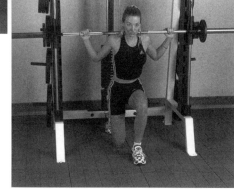

Advanced Calves Exercises

Calves are considered to be one of the most difficult muscle groups to develop. They get tremendous use when you walk or run, turn, twist, and raise up. To perform any of these movements, the calf muscles must bear all of the body's weight. Therefore, in order for the calves to respond to exercise, you must use enough weight and many specialized movements.

The primary exercise for the calves is the standing calf raise. This exercise works both the gastrocnemius and the soleus. The calves are tough and accustomed to a lot of work, so the best way to get a response from them is to shock them by using a variety of advanced training techniques described later in the chapter. You also need to subject your calves to a variety of exercise movements that will ensure complete development. Choose exercises that work each of the key areas:

Lower Calves—Seated Calf Raises

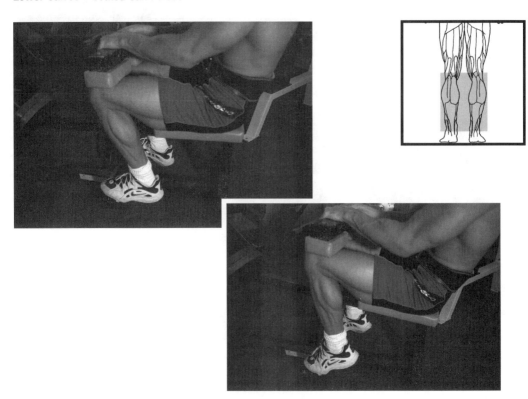

Upper Calves—Smith Machine Standing Calf Raise (with emphasis on top part of lift, hold contraction)

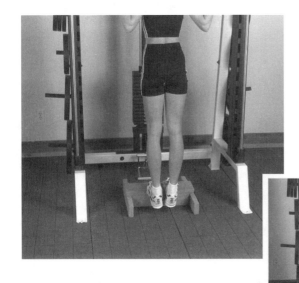

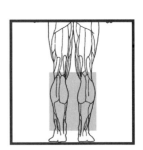

Inside Of Calves—Smith Machine Standing Calf Raises (toes pointed out)

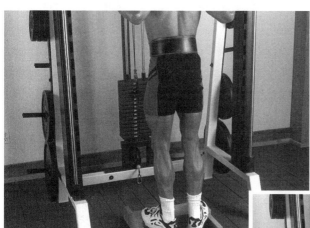
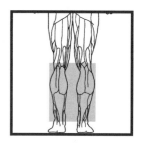
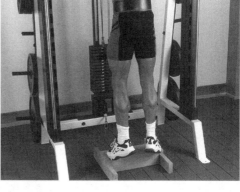

Outside Of Calves—Smith Machine Standing Calf Raises (toes pointed in)

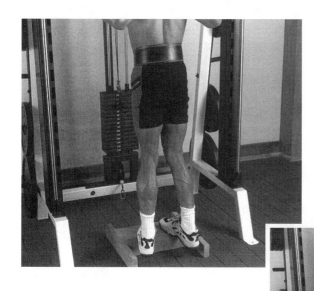
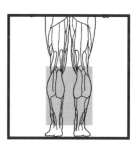

Advanced Abdomen Exercises

In order to achieve good abdominal development, consider the abdomen as four separate areas: the upper abs, lower abs, obliques, and intercostals. By working on the abdominals in this way, you can train each area as though it were an individual body part, thus ensuring proper development of all areas.

How you train your abs depends mostly on your body type. If you train the abdominal muscles with heavy weight, the muscles will become bigger and thicker. Many people actually overdevelop their abs causing them to bulge out like an inner tube around the midsection. People with small, narrow waists can enjoy success by adding weight. However, people with medium to large waists are better off not adding weight. Choose exercises that work each of the key areas:

Upper Abs—Reverse Crunches

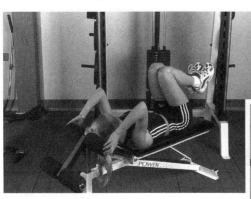
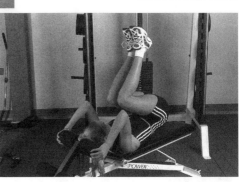

Lower Abs—Hanging Leg Raises

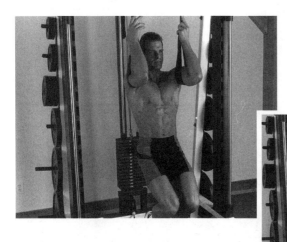
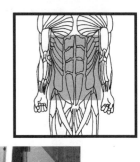

Obliques—Hanging Leg Raises (to the side)

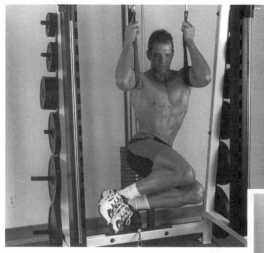
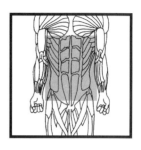
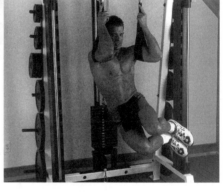

Intercostals—Broomstick Twists

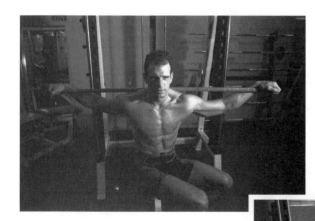
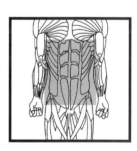

Advanced Back Exercises

To completely develop the back, you need to consider how each of the important back muscles function so that you include exercises that work all the vital areas. The key to effective back training is to isolate the key areas of the back.

Outer Back—One Arm Dumbbell Rows

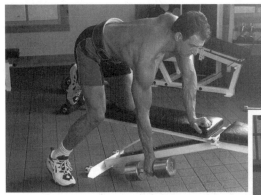
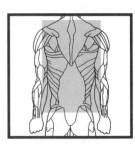
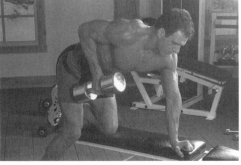

Upper Back Development—Dumbbell Reverse Upright Row

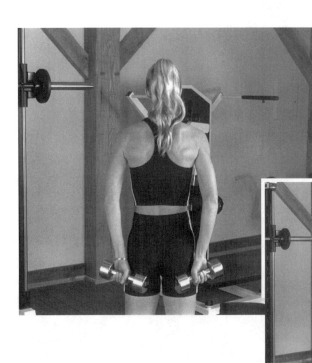
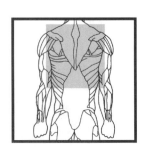

Lat Width—Wide Grip Pulldowns (front of the neck)

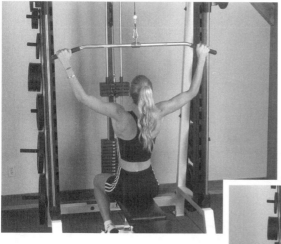
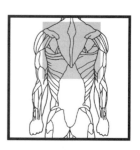
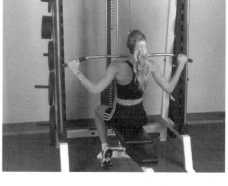

Lower Lat Development—Standing Low Pulley Row

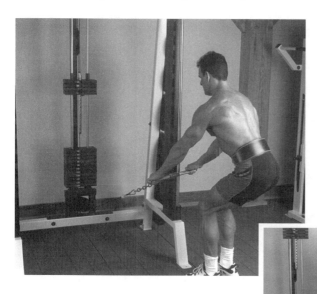
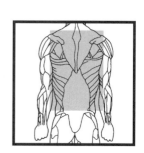

Middle Back—Stiff Arm Pulldowns

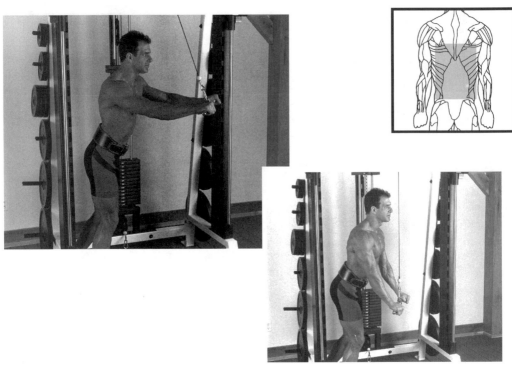

Lower Back—Smith Machine Partial Deadlifts

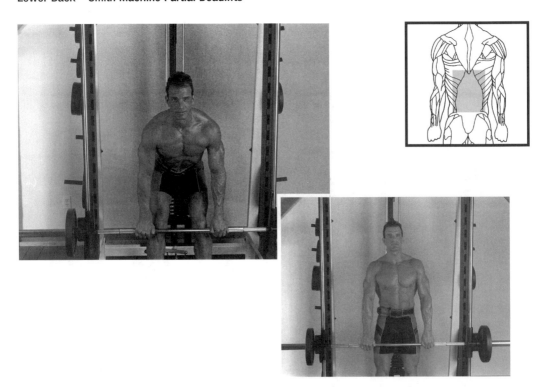

Note—Save lower back exercises until the end of the workout.

Advanced Weight Training Techniques

All the training techniques that I recommend for beginner—straight sets, circuit sets, isolation sets, progressive overload, and priority training—as well as intermediate techniques—super sets, compound sets, pyramid sets, descending sets, reverse order sets—can be used at the advanced level of training. However, there are 14 additional techniques that I consider to be good advanced level training techniques.

Giant Sets—a series of four to six exercises working one muscle group, performed with little or no rest between sets.

Burns—two or three partial reps done at the end of a regular set. Burns are good for increasing muscle size and vascularity.

Partials—good for increasing power and size. With this method, you perform only part of the movement, midpoint to finish, or start to midpoint.

Trisets—three exercises working the same muscle group, performed consecutively, with little or no rest between sets. Good for shaping, increasing definition, and vascularity.

Ten Sets Of Ten—a good technique to use when you get bored. Ten sets of ten require that you perform one set for each body part with all-out effort. Select a weight that you can use for 10 reps and do consecutive sets of 10 reps until you complete 10 sets for a total of 100 repetitions. This technique is good for shaping, increasing definition, and vascularity.

Shock Sets—when your program seems stale, shock it! Muscle eventually adapts to whatever exercise you're doing and that leads to decreasing results. Shock sets are a great way to avoid plateaus. To incorporate exercises that shock the muscle into your program, simply add exercises to your routine that you don't normally do.

Forced Reps—having a spotter help you, grind out two to three more reps after you reach a point of failure. Forced reps push your muscle fibers beyond normal fatigue to stimulate even greater growth and muscular density. This is a great technique for increasing strength/power and muscle mass. It is an intensive technique that you should use only sparingly.

Peak Contraction—keeping full tension on the working muscle or muscle group by squeezing the muscles at the end of a repetition. This technique is best for enhancing definition.

Cheat Reps—using body English to help you lift a heavier weight than you can normally lift can help you add more intensity to the lift. You can use this technique for increasing stress to a muscle and for developing strength/power and muscle mass.

Staggered Sets—performed by working smaller body parts in between larger body parts. For example, working the neck, abdominals, and forearms in between working larger body parts, such as the legs. This technique allows you to work out more efficiently by saving time.

Explosive Sets—good for sports training. You perform explosive sets by concentrating on exploding the weight on the upward or positive portion of the lift. This technique is great for increasing explosive power used in sprinting and jumping, but it's important not to use too heavy of a weight.

Rest Pause—this technique (one of my favorites) allows you to simulate very heavy lifting without using a spotter. After a set of bench presses, you rest two to three seconds and then grind out another couple of reps. You then rest for two to three more seconds and then grind out another rep or two. It is great for maximizing intensity and increasing strength/power and muscle mass.

Timed sets—a good training technique to use to improve sports performance. Grinding out as many reps as you can in a designated time will give your muscles a great pump and is an effective way to increase cardiovascular and muscular endurance. To perform this technique, do as many reps of an exercise as you can in one minute, then rest and repeat the exercise.

21's—a series of partial movements you can use when your mind and body become stale. Good for enhancing muscle definition.

Advanced Training Routines

The most common weekly training routines advanced trainees use is the split. Here are the most popular split routines.

Two-way split—2 days on, 1 off, 2 on, 2 off (over 1 week)

Day One—upper body: chest, back, shoulders, biceps, triceps
Day Two—lower body: quadriceps, hamstrings, calves
Day Three—rest
Day Four—upper body: chest, back, shoulders, biceps, triceps
Day Five—lower body: quadriceps, hamstrings, calves
Day Six—rest
Day Seven—rest

Three-way Split—3 days on, 1 off, repeat (over 1 week)

Day One—chest, shoulders, triceps
Day Two—quadriceps, hamstrings, calves
Day Three—back, biceps, forearms
Day Four—rest
Day Five—chest, shoulders, triceps
Day Six—quadriceps, hamstrings, calves
Day Seven—back, biceps, forearms

Four-way split—4 days on, 1 off, (modified, this is the program I use)

Day One—chest, calves, abdominals
Day Two—shoulder, triceps, abdominals
Day Three—quadriceps, hamstrings, abdominals
Day Four—back, biceps, forearms, abdominals
Day Five—rest
Day Six—start the sequence over

Cycle Your Training

Training at the advanced level will require maximum effort and intensity. You should practice periodization, dividing your training schedule into cycles.

Cycling your training is very important at the advanced level because the demands of training will take their toll and will require some rest periods. Without periods of rest your body will burn out, experience aches, pains, and progress can be halted.

Sets And Reps

At this level you should perform three to four sets per exercise for the upper body, four to six sets for the legs, and three to six sets for the abdomen. Your goals will determine the number of reps. For example, if your goal is to train for strength/power/mass, you should perform one to six repetitions. For general muscle tone, you should perform 8 to 12 repetitions, and for muscular endurance perform 12 to 25 repetitions.

Rest Between Sets

If your goal is to build strength/power/mass, you should rest two to four minutes; for muscle tone (definition, shape, vascularity) rest one to two minutes, and for muscular endurance rest 30 seconds to one minute between sets.

Stretching

Stretching is very important at the advanced level. You should begin stretching the muscle you have just worked after completing each set. Perform the basic stretches outlined in Chapter Nine. Stretching between sets is a great way to enhance the muscle pump, as well as defining and shaping the muscle. Always remember to stretch before, during, and after your training.

Chapter 13
Training For Safe Weight Loss

In today's fast-food world you may be faced with the same challenge that many people face—too much body fat. I have been on this side of the coin more than once. I have probably lost close to over 200 pounds in my lifetime. For years I played the yo-yo game of gain weight, lose weight. When I was a junior in high school, I weighed 235 pounds. As a sophomore in college, I weighed 250 pounds. You can bet that I know just how you feel. I truly understand your desires to improve yourself. After I lost the weight, it made a drastic difference in my self-esteem. I felt better about myself, tripled my energy, and was a much happier person.

We all know that being overweight can be a hazard to our overall health. Today, it seems every year more and more people are reported as being overweight and out-of-shape. And the major cause—high fat, processed food diets combined with inactivity.

Taking charge of your nutritional habits is a must. After all, evidence shows us that it doesn't get any easier as we get older.

Warning—Weight Loss Can Be Hazardous To Your Health
Going on a diet, cutting back calories, losing weight, and changing the shape of the body is serious business. I have seen people who attempted this in unhealthy ways wind up in the hospital, suffer from eating disorders, cause permanent damage to their bodies, become depressed, even die from misguided, unhealthy practices of losing weight.

There is only one way to safely and effectively lose weight—stick to a good nutrition, exercise, and training program.

Forget what the ads say, forget about the magic potions, products, and pills.

Weight Loss and Body Shaping Training Program
It's pretty hard to tell someone who wants to lose a lot of weight to exercise three times per week, eat a sensible diet, and wait for the results to appear. When I was attempting to lose 50 pounds, I knew that that approach was not going to work for me. So I experimented and I discovered a workout that gave me fantastic results. By following it I was able to trim 50 pounds of body fat while at the same time toning, strengthening, and shaping my body.

I trained five days in a row, dividing the body up over five sessions. Each session consisted of weight training one major body part, abdominal training, and some form of aerobic conditioning. I followed this schedule Monday through Friday taking the weekends off for rest. I did not, however, veg out and sit on the couch all weekend. I usually did some form of recreational activity like riding my bike or playing basketball.

Weight Loss Training Routine
Monday—chest, abs, aerobic training
Tuesday—shoulders, abs, fat burning training
Wednesday—back, abs, aerobic training
Thursday—arms, abs, fat burning
Friday—legs, abs, aerobic training

Monday—Smith Machine Chest Press

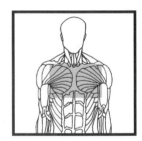

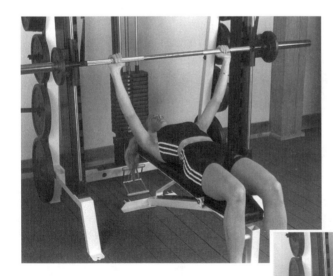

Incline Dumbbell Press

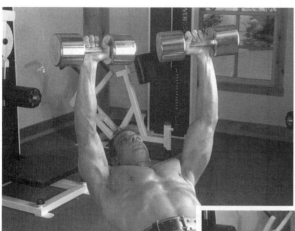
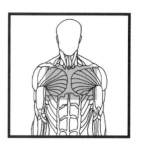
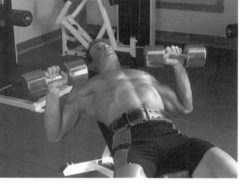

Dumbbell Flat Bench Flys

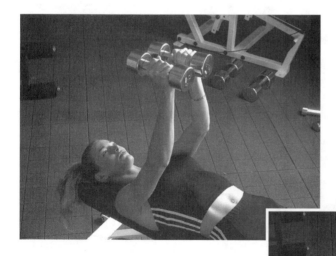
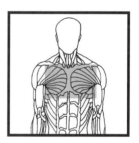

Smith Machine Decline Press

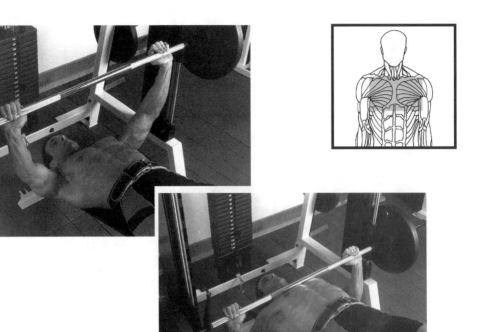

Crunch

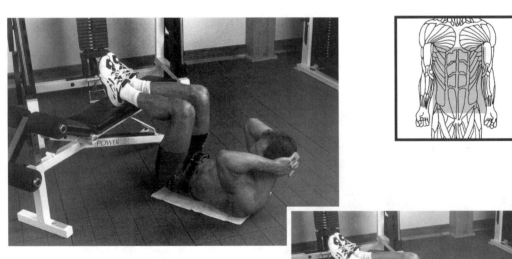

Seated Leg Raise

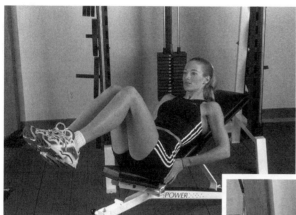
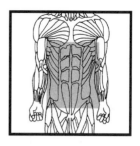
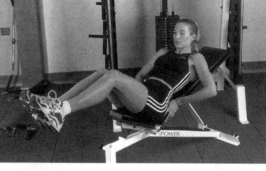

Tuesday—Smith Machine Shoulder Press

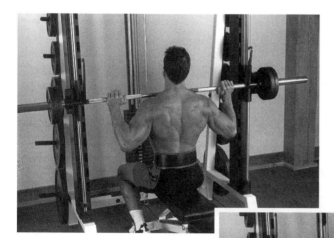
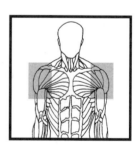

Dumbbell Shoulder Press

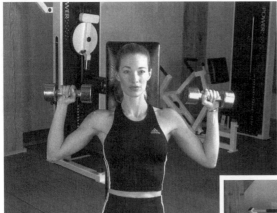
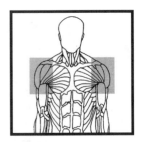
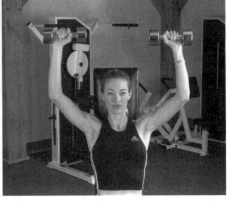

Barbell Upright Row

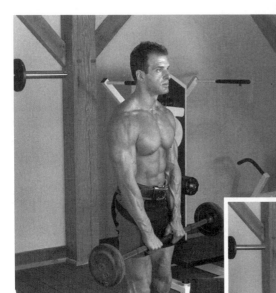
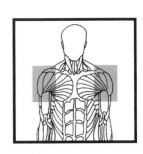

Dumbbell Front Raise

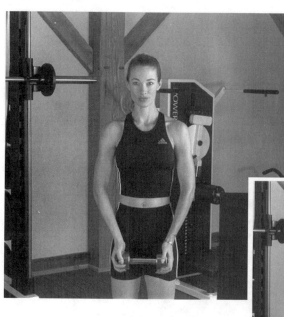
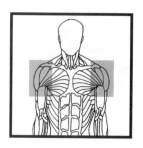
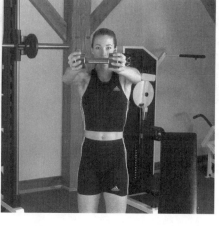

Cable Crunch

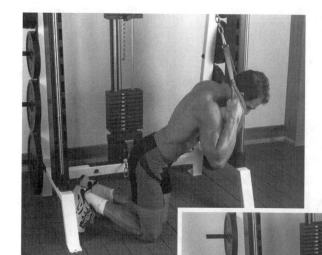
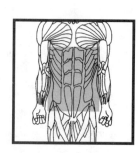

Hanging Leg Raise

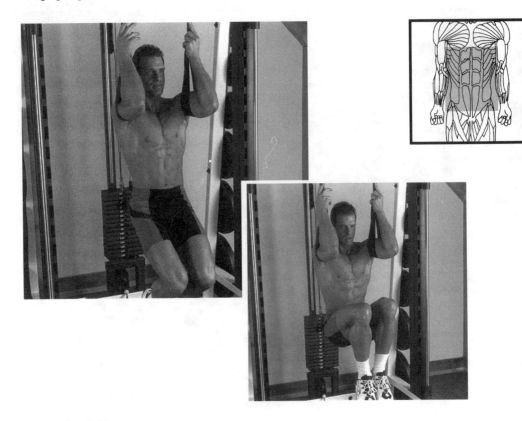

Broomstick Twists

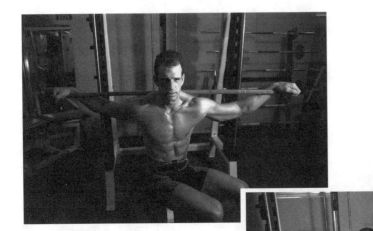

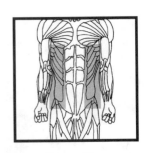

Wednesday—Lat Machine Pulldown

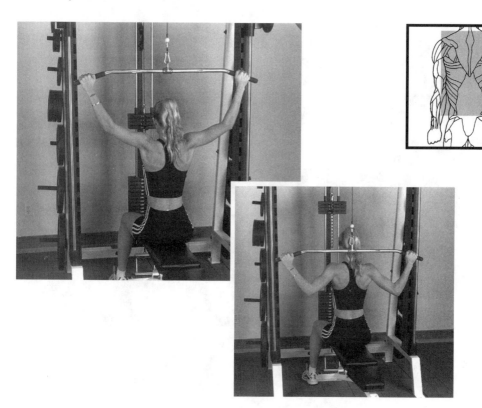

Seated Low Pulley Row

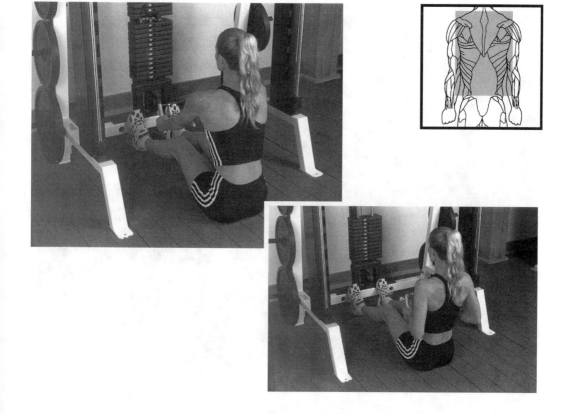

Reverse Smith Upright Row

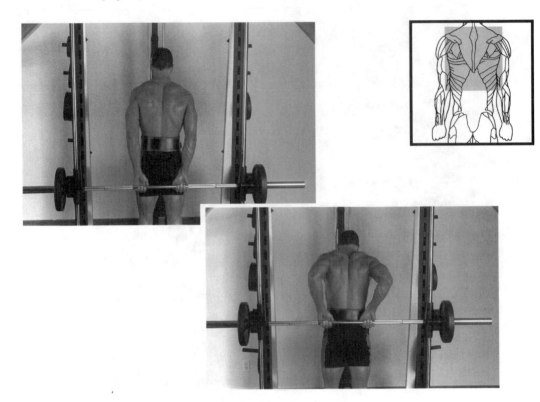

Hyperextension

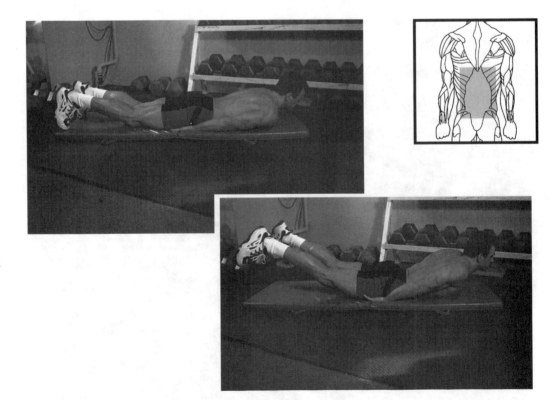

Incline Partial Sit-up

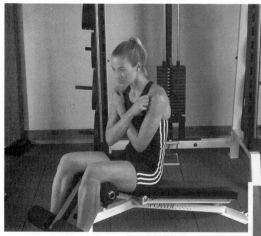
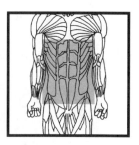
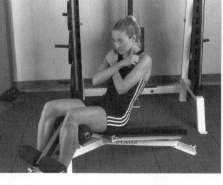

Reverse Crunch

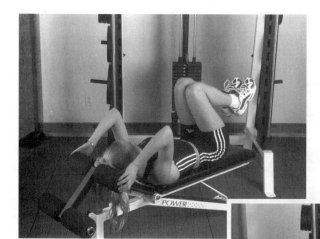
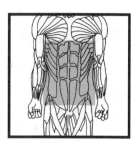

Thursday—Barbell Arm Curl

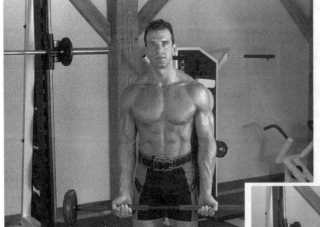
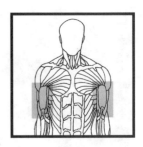
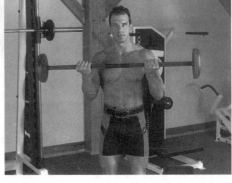

Dumbbell Hammer Curl

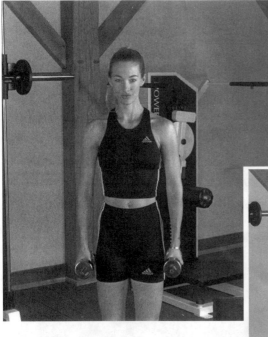
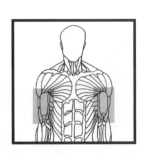
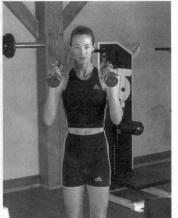

Smith Machine Close Grip Press

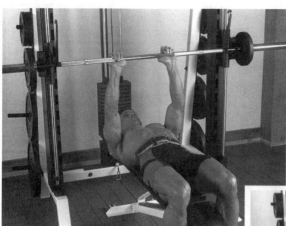
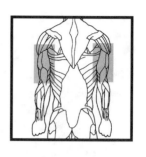
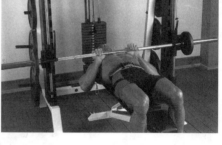

Bench Dips

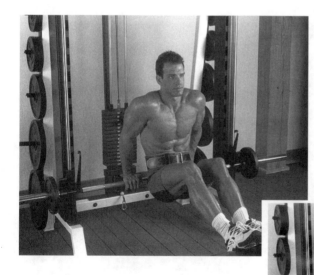
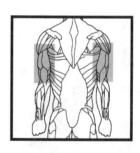

Crunches

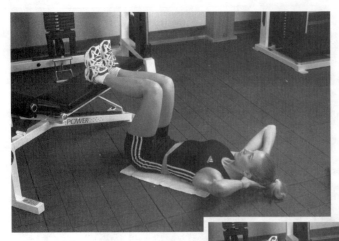
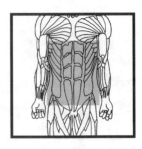

Incline Knee-ups

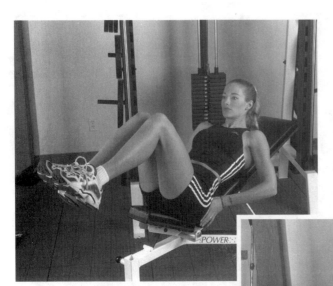
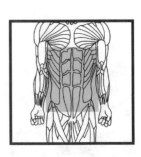

Friday—Leg Press

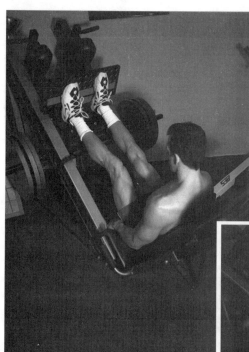
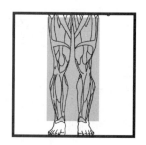
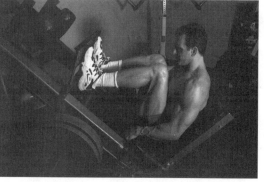

Smith Machine Squat

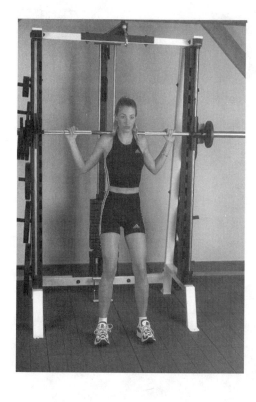
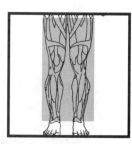
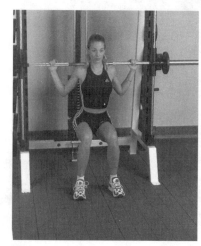

Leg Extension

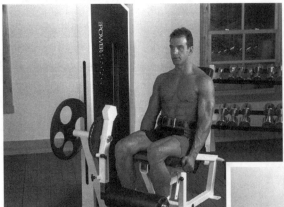
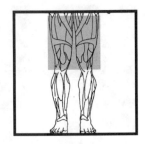
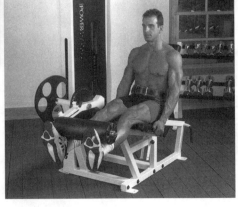

Leg Curl

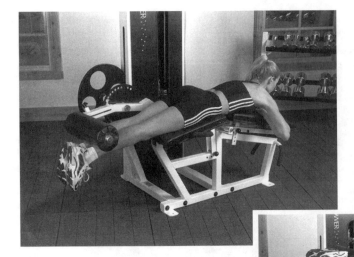
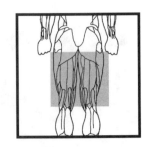

Smith Machine Standing Calf Raise

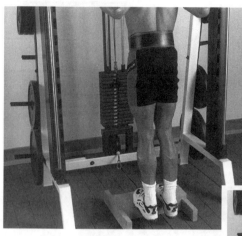
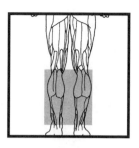
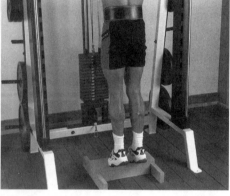

Seated Calf Raise

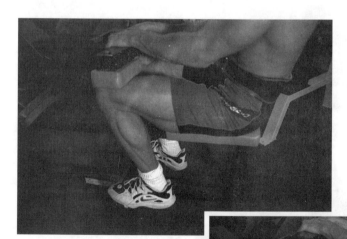
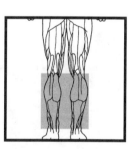

Reverse Crunch

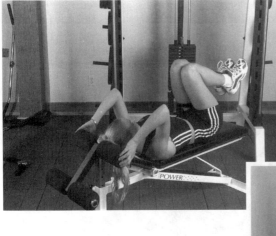
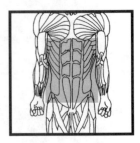
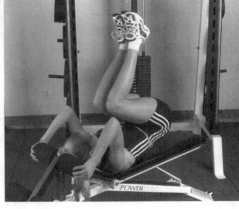

Hanging Leg Raise

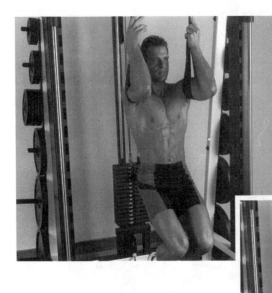
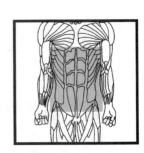

Weight Loss Sets And Reps

1st exercise on each day
1st set 12 reps
2nd set 8 reps
3rd set 6 reps

2nd and consecutive exercises
1st set 10 reps
2nd set 8 reps

Weight Loss Poundages

All Upper Body Exercises
Increase weight 5-10 lbs. per set

Lower Body Exercises—Leg Press, Squat, Calf Raise
Increase weight 10-20 lbs. per set

Leg Extension And Leg Curl
Increase weight 5-10 lbs. per set

Nonweight Assisted Exercises—Abdominals and Hyperextensions
Exercise to failure

Rest Between Sets

1-2 minutes

Techniques

Pyramid—Increase the weight for each set while at the same time decreasing the number of reps you perform.

Aerobic Training

Monday after weights
Jog, treadmill, stationary bike, or row, etc.
20 minutes with heart rate in the 75% range

Tuesday after weights
Jog, treadmill, stationary bike, or row, etc.
35 minutes with heart rate in the 65% range

Wednesday after weights
Jog, treadmill, stationary bike, or row, etc.
45 minutes with heart rate in the 55% range

Thursday after weights
Jog, treadmill, stationary bike, or row, etc.
15 minutes with heart rate in the 75% range

Friday after weights
Jog, treadmill, stationary bike, or row, etc.
30 minutes with heart rate in the 60% range

Stretching

Full body stretch after all weight training and aerobic workouts.

(See Chapter Nine for key body stretches.)

Special Training Notes

Remember the goal is to safely lose body fat. Include these guidelines in your program:

* Shoot to lose no more than two pounds a week, preferably one pound a week
* Get body fat tested, find out lean body mass
* Chart and monitor your weight loss, weighing in twice a week
* Include supplements in your diet (see Chapter Twenty-Eight)
* Get plenty of rest
* Don't use rubber suits to "sweat it out"

Sometimes it happens—you overexercise and diet to excess. Here are the warning signs:

* Irritability
* Loss of appetite
* Dizziness/lightheadedness
* Loss of focus, concentration
* Continued loss of weight
* Weakness
* Soft muscles

* Losing more than 3-4 pounds a week

Nutrition And Weight Loss

What you put into your mouth is going to determine about 70 percent of your success while on a weight loss program. As the saying goes, "You can out eat any exercise program." Work in the gym is a given, but you will have to work equally hard on your nutritional program in order to succeed. You will have to learn:

* The basics of nutrition (see Chapter Six)
* How foods affect your body
* How to prepare meals
* When to eat
* What to eat
* Where to eat
* Why you should eat.
* Supplements, vitamins, and minerals

Set Up A System Of Checks And Balances

Most people who are concerned with their weight don't need fancy body fat tests to tell them when they are overweight. Most see it in the mirror and feel the effects. I know this all too well myself. As a junior in high school, I weighed 235 pounds I didn't need a test to tell me. I saw my stomach sticking out in the mirror and felt bloated, fatigued, and unmotivated.

However, I think it is a good idea to get tested if possible to see what your body fat percentage is and to periodically get tested during your training and weight loss program.

Safe, effective weight loss is a lot more than just lowering the numbers on the scale. There is a huge difference between losing body fat and losing muscle mass. One of the first things you need to learn about both weight loss and weight gain is the difference between lean muscle mass and body fat.

Good Ways To Safely Gauge Weight Loss

There are informal methods: photographs, videotaping, tape measures, and scales. These are easy to use and require little time and effort. I feel they are probably the most practical for nearly everyone.

Scientific methods include muscular fitness tests, cardiovascular fitness tests, and body composition analysis. These offer a more scientific measurement of your progress and seem to appeal to people who are more statistically minded and like cold, hard facts.

Photographs are my favorite method of measuring my progress because they allow me to see my body as it really is. With photographs, you can get a 360 degree view of your body, providing a realistic perspective on how it looks from every angle. Photographs also give you a permanent record of what your body looked like at a specific time.

The easiest, quickest, least time-consuming and most economical way to gauge your progress is to simply look in the mirror. The mirror gives us the opportunity to catch a glimpse of our progress any time we wish. I recommend using the mirror for day-to-day feedback. It's a pretty good judgment of your actual progress.

However, there are some drawbacks with using the mirror as a gauging tool. It is only natural to focus on what we want to see. Some people focus on the good areas. Whereas, others will not see their progress because they can't get past looking at the areas that haven't changed shape. Another problem is that unless you are able to purchase a special three-way mirror or set up a series of mirrors, you will only be able to see a limited view of yourself.

The tape measure is a popular method for gauging progress because it gives a reading of your body size. A scale can give you total pounds lost or gained, but the tape measure precisely provides the size of each area of your body.

The Key Points To Follow When Using A Tape Measure

* Use the same tape measure every time
* Use a cloth tape measure—plastic tape measures eventually stretch and won't give accurate measurements
* Have the same person measure you each time
* Record all measurements to the closest sixteenth of an inch. Take measurements before working out
* Relax your muscles while they are being measured
* Take measurements in the middle of the muscle
* Don't pull the tape too tight or let it hang too loose
* Always measure the same area

Twelve key measurements to take:
* Neck
* Biceps (right and left)
* Forearm (right and left)
* Chest
* Waist
* Hips
* Thighs (right and left)
* Calves (right and left)

I like to use measurements to determine if the body is losing weight evenly throughout. However, tape measurements can be very misleading if you only pay attention to inches lost or gained. Measurements can't show whether you're losing muscle mass or body fat. They can only denote that a change has occurred.

The scale is probably the most widely used piece of equipment for gauging progress. Unfortunately, it is the most misleading and inaccurate. Scales do not make a distinction between body fat and lean muscle mass. So if the scale shows you have lost 10 pounds, have you lost 10 pounds of muscle mass or body fat? Body fat weighs less than muscle mass. Therefore, when you weigh five pounds more yet measure inches smaller, have you gained or lost? My best advice is to throw away your scale!

If you're like most people on any training program, you want to increase your lean body mass and decrease your body fat. It is possible to gauge your progress in this area by monitoring your body composition. Sophisticated tests can tell you how much lean body mass and how much body fat you have. All of the available methods used for this type of measurement require a different level of commitment, time, and expense, and offer varying degrees of accuracy. None of the tests are perfect, although some are better than others.

The best body composition analysis test is the hydrostatic or underwater weighing analysis. This method is considered to be 98 percent accurate. Hydrostatic body composition analysis must be performed by a special technician in a special dunk tank, and usually costs $50 to $100.

The caliper test (skin fold) is the most popular method for gauging body composition. This method, used by colleges, sports teams, and health clubs should be performed by a knowledgeable technician. The results are found by taking about seven skin fold measurements from various parts of the body. The technician then manipulates these numbers according to a formula to determine your approximate body fat percentage. Though this method has proven effective over the years, it is only as accurate as the operator administering it. So check out the technician's credentials, and try to use the same person for your test each time.

These tests may seem rather elaborate for something most of us can do just by looking in the mirror and being honest with ourselves. However, athletes, bodybuilders, and fitness enthusiasts have used body composition analysis for years to ensure their success. Yet many others who have not taken advantage of these tests have reached the same success levels of those who have. Whether you choose to use these tests as a gauge of your progress is strictly up to you.

Chapter 14
Training For Fat-Free Weight Gain

Although this may be hard for many people to believe, there are those rare individuals who struggle with putting on weight just like those who struggle to take off weight. Today, it is hard for me to believe that after spending more than half my life training to lose weight and keep from gaining weight, that I now have to work very hard to keep my weight from dropping. My system has become so efficient and tuned up that I can easily lose weight. Because my body fat level is so low, when I lose weight now it is usually muscle mass—the weight that is not good to lose. When I talk about putting on weight, I am not referring to getting fat. I mean putting on quality weight—lean muscle mass—opposed to body fat.

Many people make the mistake of thinking that eating everything in sight is the way to gain weight or bulk up. Weight gain is only good if it is quality muscle mass.

The safest way to put on weight is gradually. The most I like to shoot for is about a pound or two every two weeks. This doesn't sound like much but a pound every two weeks is two pounds a month, which equals 24 pounds a year. That's a lot!

Even gaining one pound a month doesn't seem like much, but when you add it up, it's a total of 12 pounds a year. Keep in mind that as an adult a 10-pound weight gain over the course of a year can drastically alter your appearance.

There are three important areas of consideration when training for weight gain: weight training, nutrition, and recovery.

Training Programs for Weight Gain

A consistent weight training program is essential to gaining quality, lean muscle mass. Weight training is the way you build muscle. And muscle is the quality weight that you want to gain. The best routines for gaining weight are those that involve basic movements, such as:

* Bench Press
* Seated Row
* Shoulder Press
* Squats
* Leg Press

In other words, you're going to have to train hard in the weight room.

Training Routine

Monday—Heavy Upper Body
chest, back, shoulders, biceps, triceps, neck, abs

Tuesday—Heavy Lower Body
quadriceps, hamstrings, calves, lower back, abs

Thursday—Light Upper Body
chest, back, shoulders, biceps, triceps, neck, abs

Friday—Light Lower Body
quadriceps, hamstrings, calves, lower back, abs

Monday/Thursday—Barbell Chest Press

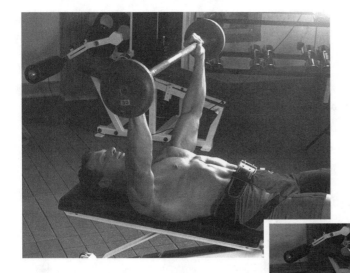
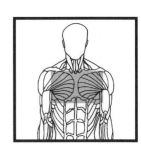

Incline Dumbbell Press

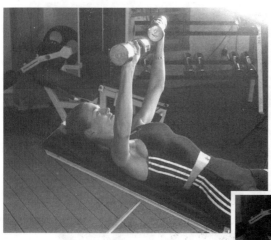
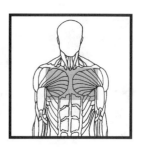
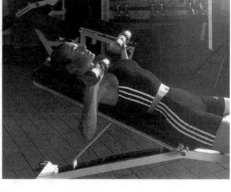

Lat Pulldown Wide Grip (behind the neck)

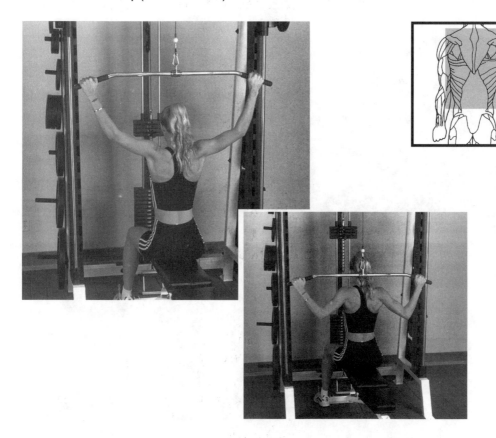

Seated Low Pulley Cable Row

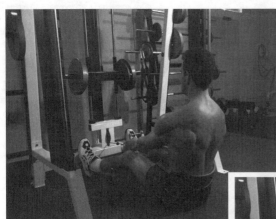
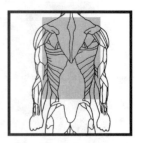
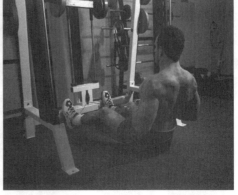

Smith Machine Shoulder Press (front of neck)

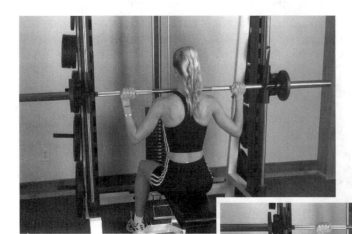
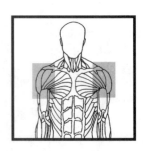

Barbell Upright Row

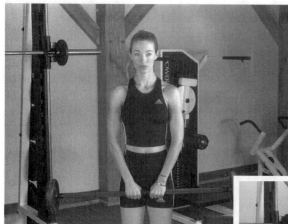
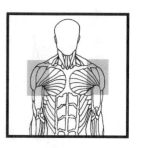
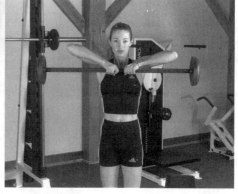

Smith Machine Shoulder Shrug

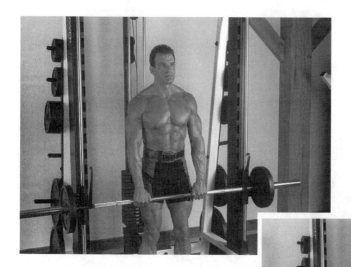
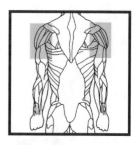

Barbell Arm Curl

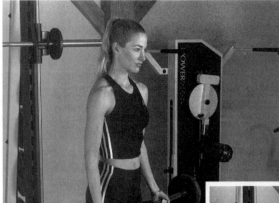
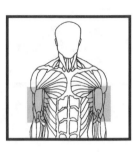
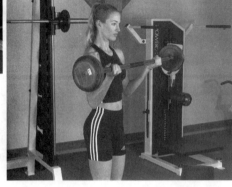

Bench Dips

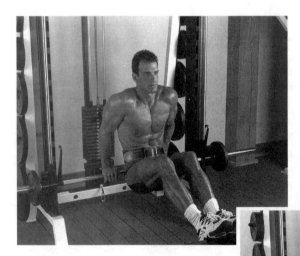
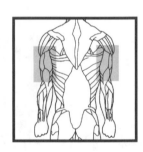

Partial Incline Sit-Up

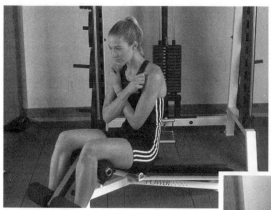
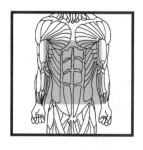
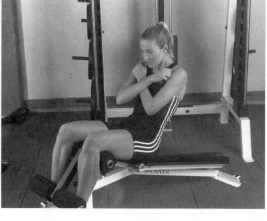

Hanging Leg Raise

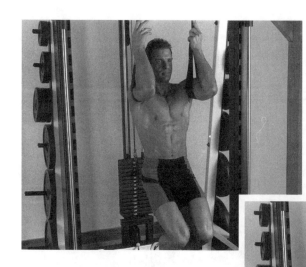
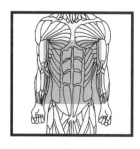

Tuesday/Thursday—Leg Press

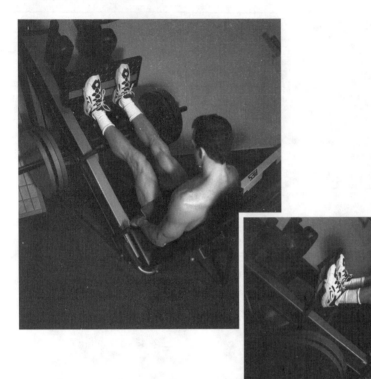

Smith Machine Squat

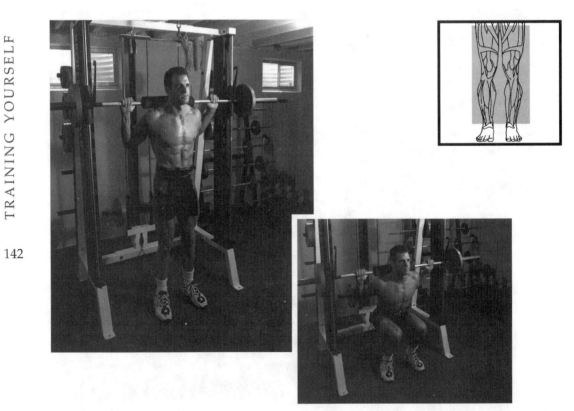

Leg Extension

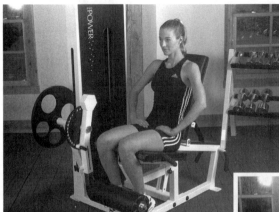
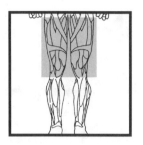
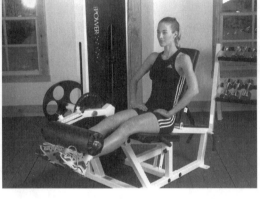

Lying Leg Curl

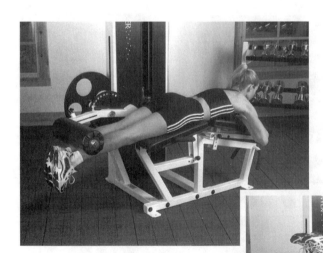
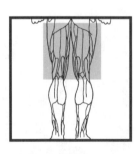

Smith Machine Standing Calf Raise

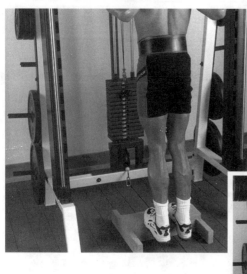
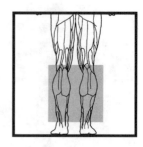
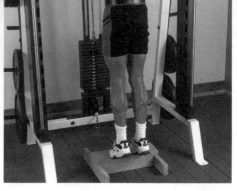

Crunch

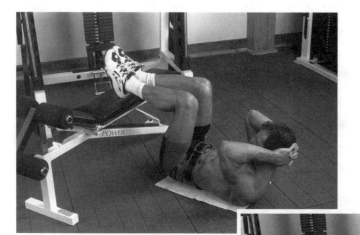
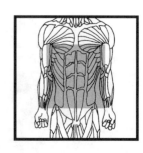

Incline Bench Knee-Ups

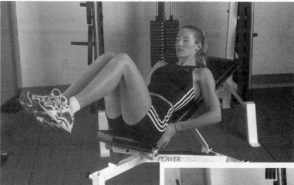
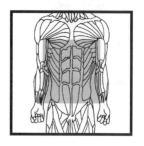
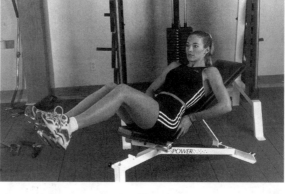

Hyperextension

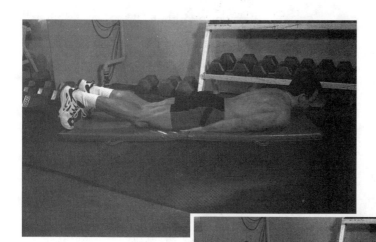
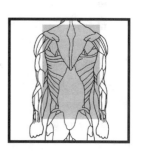

Sets & Reps

Monday/Tuesday—Heavy Day

3 sets of each exercise

1st set 10 reps, 2nd set 8 reps, 3rd set 6 reps

Thursday/Friday—Light Day

2 sets of each exercise

1st set 12 reps, 2nd set 8 reps

Poundages

All Upper Body Exercises

Increase weight 5-10 lbs. per set

Lower Body Exercises — Leg Press, Squat, Calf Raise

Increase weight 10-20 lbs. per set

Leg Extension and Leg Curl

Increase weight 5-10 lbs. per set

Nonweight Assisted Exercises—Neck Isos, Abdominals, Hyperextensions

Exercise to failure

Rest Between Sets

2 minutes

Aerobic Training

Traditionally most people engage in aerobic exercise to lose weight—"burn off the fat." However, aerobic exercise is also important for those who want to gain weight.

According to some experts, aerobic exercise builds cardiovascular density which means it increases the size and number of blood vessels in your circulatory system. This enables more nutrients to be transported to all body tissues, including your muscles.

Aerobic exercise also increases total blood volume, which flushes toxins from your body more quickly. This results in less fatigue and an ability for your muscles to recover more quickly following strenuous exercise.

Using the following program, I was able to get great results. It involves three aerobic training sessions over the course of a week. Two jogging days and one day of sprints. I found that by adding a day of sprint work, my legs developed much better and my strength and power increased quite a bit.

Workout 1	Jog 30 minutes
Workout 2	Run 20 minutes (hustle pace)
Workout 3	Sprints or strides on treadmill

Stretching

Full body stretch after all weight training and aerobic workouts. (See Chapter Nine for key body stretches.)

Nutrition

Nutrition means eating the right combination of foods along with a good supplementation program. Nutrition is a primary factor in recovering from training. Physical training requires proper nutrition in order to ensure that your body is getting all of the vital nutrients it needs to recover from intense training.

The keys to nutrition anD weight gain are:

Get enough protein—Proteins are essential for growth and maintenance of all body tissue. Proteins serve as a major source of building material for muscle, blood, skin, hair, and nails, and for the internal organs, primarily the heart and brain. Proteins also produce hormones that regulate a host of bodily functions, including metabolic rates and antibodies that combat foreign substances in the body.

Take your supplements—Supplements are like insurance. They're there when you need them. Supplements are a great way to ensure that your body is getting all the nutrients it needs to recover and grow from training. Preparing foods, cooking, and processing all destroy valuable nutrients. Taking supplements is a way to ensure that your body has a good supply of nutrients on hand when it needs it.

Eat four to six small higher protein meals throughout the day—Keeping your body fed throughout the day is a good way to keep it loaded with the nutrients it needs to function properly. Starving the body causes it to stress. When the body is stressed it doesn't recover and grow.

Try to eat a nutritional meal before you go to bed—Eating a small meal before you go to bed will ensure that your body has the nutrients it needs to go through the recovery process as you sleep. My favorite is a protein shake just before turning in.

Don't eat junk food thinking that it will help you gain good weight—Just because you need to gain weight does not mean you should eat everything in sight. Remember, the goal of weight gain training is to put on quality weight—lean muscle mass. Loading up on processed empty calorie foods will definitely cause you to gain weight—in body fat!

What about weight gain powders? Weight gain powders are a popular item sold in many nutrition stores. But I question the value of many of them. Most are loaded with sugars—and too much sugar makes you fat. You want to gain good weight, solid lean muscle mass, not body fat. I have found it better to supplement with good protein powder and recovery formula.

Recovery

The mental and physical demands of training place special importance on recovery factors. In weight training, the muscles do not increase in size until after they have thoroughly recovered from your preceding workout. Muscles grow during the resting phase of training, not during the actual lifting. The important recovery factors are:

Smart Training + Nutrition + Rest = Results

Training is only a part of the equation. Training too hard, too long, and too often is not going to allow your body to grow. Overtraining can even cause you to tear your muscles down rather then build them up.

Smart training means getting the most results from the least amount of effort. I am not suggesting that you not put a lot of effort into your workout. You must train with intensity. Merely going through the motions will get you nowhere. Just don't forget that you must also take time off for your muscles to recover.

Muscle Soreness

When you train with intensity, your muscles will become mildly sore for a day or two after you exercise them. They won't be sore in the way they were when you first began training. As crazy as it sounds, the soreness you will experience will be a comfortable sensation. It is a feeling that you will actually learn to look forward to. If your muscles don't become sore, then you will know that you haven't pushed yourself hard enough. And if that's the case, you will need to reevaluate your training program. If you are constantly sore, then you are getting too much of a good thing. Soreness is the result of micro tears in the muscle fibers. These tears at the cellular level are repaired as the muscles grow. If you exercise so much that your body is always sore, you never give your muscles the time they need to grow stronger. A good rule of thumb to follow in recovery is to never exercise a body part until it has been free from soreness for at least a day.

Rest

Rest is also a vital part of the recovery process. We all know that the body requires rest to perform at its best. This includes adequate sleep and enough relaxation time during our waking hours to bring about a state of physical and mental refreshment. Many of the benefits derived from sleep actually occur in the first few hours of the sleeping state. It is during this period that most people fall into a deep sleep during which the repair process operates at full speed. The greatest release of growth hormone also takes place during these first few hours.

Different people have different sleep requirements. Some people can get along on as little as five or six hours, while others require at least eight hours of restful sleep.

The body also performs at its best when sleep takes place at roughly the same time every night. This programmed timetable provides a continuity the body thrives on.

Recovery means paying attention to:
- Time off
- Sleep
- Stress management
- Rest
- Lay offs
- Nutrition
- Training

Chapter 15
Injury and Overtraining

Training seriously for 20 years, as well as participating in 12 years of competitive sports, you can bet I have had my share of injuries. I've had two knee surgeries, bouts with a nasty sciatica, rotator cuff damage in my right shoulder, and about 14 bouts of pinched nerves in my lower back.

In all likelihood, if you're training or participating in recreational sports, there is a good chance the you will suffer from an injury at some time or another.

Most injuries are not devastating. With proper rest, combined with good rehabilitation and nutrition, you will mend in no time at all.

Training Injuries

There are many types of injuries you might encounter in training and sports. There are injuries to muscles, bones, tendons, and ligaments which usually occur as strains, sprains, dislocations, fractures, and breaks.

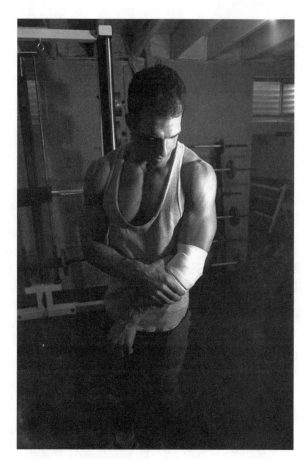

The obvious serious injuries like breaks, fractures, dislocations, and severe strains and sprains require immediate medical attention. That's the only solution. Do not ever attempt to self-remedy a serious injury.

For the most part, most training injuries are muscle related and are not severe enough to warrant medical attention. These injuries often occur for several reasons:

* Improper or no warm-up
* Lack of flexibility
* Reaching beyond current conditioning/overstraining
* Overloading an unhealed injury
* Underdeveloped muscle or muscles
* Carelessness
* Poor technique or skill execution
* Overtraining

Most muscle injuries can be self-treated. Ice and heat treatments, light training or light rehabilitation exercises, and rest, along with good supplementation will have you back to training in no time.

Remember for severe injuries like tendon and ligament injuries, play it safe and see a doctor.

For Your Mental Attitude

Injuries not only put a strain on you physically, but they can be mentally painful or stressful as well. Many report that during injuries they experience:

* Depression
* Loss of motivation
* Frustration
* Anxiety
* Loss of appetite

Injuries are a part of high intensity training. The mental outlook you have on injuries will make the difference in your ability to deal with the setbacks and the time off for rehabilitation. I know that it's disappointing to be going along, making really good progress, and then to have it halted because of a nagging injury.

But injuries don't have to be a time of gloom and despair. Time off for injuries can be a positive and productive time. With the right attitude, you can use the time wisely to improve the other aspects of your training. You can:

* Develop the mental side of your training
* Use the time to train the rest of your body
* Work on becoming more aerobically fit
* Reevaluate your training program
* Overhaul your diet

What You Can Do To Avoid Injuries

Prevention is the best medicine. This can be done in many ways. Conditioning — getting in good shape and staying there. Keeping personal stress levels down. Get plenty of rest. I always recommend at least eight hours of sleep. Learn to train, relaxed and in control. This is accomplished through hours and hours of practice. Eat a healthy diet and take supplements. Always warm up and stretch prior to training.

Overtraining

You would think that if a little training is good then a lot of training would be better. It seems logical.

But in training, it's a little different. Sometimes more is not better. Sometimes more is actually less.

Exercise and training all break the body down. In weight training for instance, when you curl a dumbbell, you actually damage the muscle fibers of the arm. As a matter of fact, they don't grow, or get stronger, until they have rested and rebuilt themselves. The results come after the training, in the rest phase.

Training the body too hard or too often does not allow it to recover and forces it into a state called overtraining. It's a damaging state which creates muscle loss, drains energy, and lowers the immune system.

Probably the biggest culprit of injuries in training is overtraining. This can occur for many reasons: doing too much too soon, not getting enough rest, a poor diet, and a poorly designed training program.

To be successful with your training, it's important that you learn the signs of overtraining and how to combat it if it happens to you. In all likelihood, if you're training hard, you will experience it at some time. It's important that you heed the warning signs of overtraining so you can take the appropriate actions to rectify it.

Common Signs of Overtraining

* Loss of appetite
* Irritability
* Lack of motivation
* Excessive muscle soreness, aches, and pains
* Nagging injury
* Loss of body weight
* Illness—colds, flu, etc.
* Decrease in performance
* Significant loss of strength

When overtraining occurs, it's best to immediately take measures to counter it. Usually by making immediate changes in your training routine, diet, and rest patterns, you can eliminate the symptoms quickly and easily.

How To Combat Overtraining

Change your training routine
Get extra rest
Take a day off from training
Cut your training time down
Take extra supplements
Increase your quality food intake

Conclusion

Injuries are a part of being physically active. Some injuries are serious and can require immediate medical attention. Others are not so serious and can be treated using ice, heat, and rest.

Overtraining is when you train too hard and too often. The warning signs indicate that immediate changes need to be made to your routine, diet, and rest schedule.

Remember the best medicine for injuries is prevention. If an injury occurs, get immediate treatment. Learn to recognize the signs of overtraining and you will have a long training career.

Good Rule: work with training discomfort, but never work through pain!

Chapter 16
Training And Pregnancy

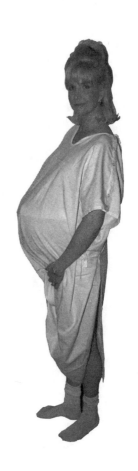

A Word Of Caution

As you read through this chapter and Chapter 17, please keep in mind that I am sharing this information with you so YOU CAN USE IT TO MAKE INTELLIGENT TRAINING DECISIONS ACCORDING TO YOUR OWN SITUATION. In no way am I saying that you should do exactly what we did, nor am I saying that this is the only way. You will have to make your own decisions on how you are going to approach training and pregnancy. No one can really tell you, "This is the program you must follow." You have to take that responsibility. Training during pregnancy is somewhat controversial. That is why it is so hard for professionals to come out and say, "This is the only way you should train during pregnancy."

My goal in these chapters is to share with you what we did. Hopefully you can take the information and say, "This might work for me," or, "I can use this part." You can take the information and mold it into your own training program. I'm not going to make specific recommendations or give you a specific program to follow. Instead, I want to show what we did and how we were able to enhance the pregnancy process, speed recovery, and achieve optimum post-pregnancy results.

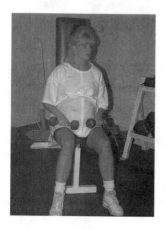

When my wife, Angela, became pregnant, she was very concerned about what pregnancy was going to do to her body. She had been training for several years and had achieved great results. I suspect her concern was one every woman gets when she becomes pregnant. It is a valid concern because for many women pregnancy is the point when they begin to face a host of physical challenges, including excessive weight gain, loss of muscle shape and tone, and the development of poor nutritional habits. How many times have you heard a woman say, "My body lost its shape after I had a baby"?

We decided to use this opportunity to conduct a real-life study of pregnancy and training. Since, as a male, I could never experience pregnancy, I felt this was as close as I could come to learning how to train my female clients through their pregnancies.

Over the course of the pregnancy, we experimented and developed a program that satisfied Angela's desire to stay in shape, was easy to perform, and protected the safety of the baby. I knew we would learn a lot about training during pregnancy, but I didn't realize how much.

A New Twist To The Pregnancy Training Experiment

Angela's pregnancy went very well. We were blessed with a healthy son and Angela quickly bounced back to her pre-pregnancy condition. Soon she was back to her normal training routine, and I thought our experiment was over.

However, 18 months later...That's right, Angela was pregnant a second time.

I felt like this presented another great opportunity to experiment by changing the variables. We had already learned how to train with pregnancy, but what about proving that training was beneficial to pregnancy in general? Angela had exercised through her first pregnancy, but how would her body respond to pregnancy without the exercise? Would it be better? Worse? The same? We decided to find out. Throughout the second pregnancy, Angela did not train at all! We documented the results and compared them with the first pregnancy.

I was excited about what I had learned from Angela's pregnancies and began to write a book about our experiment. We came up with the title *Baby Fat*. I had completed a large chunk of the book, the cover had been designed, and a marketing plan was being formed. Then one of my clients became pregnant. She wanted me to

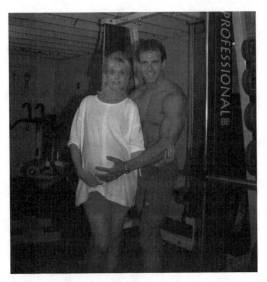

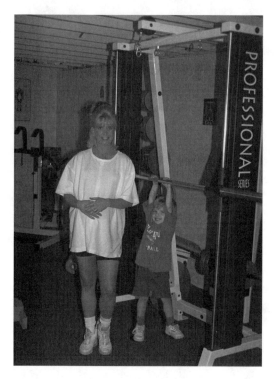

train her through the pregnancy and help her get back into shape after the baby was born. Due to my schedule, I was unable to work with her. By the fourth or fifth month of her pregnancy, we had not been able to coordinate a single training session. I felt like I had missed an opportunity to share what I had learned during Angela's pregnancies. Then in the client's fifth month of pregnancy, she lost the baby.

I was shaken. The event made me think twice about the book. I kept thinking, "If I had been training her during this time, it's very likely that I would have been blamed for exercising her too hard."

I worried that people would have rushed to judgment and unfairly accused the training as the cause of the miscarriage. As you can imagine, a situation like that could turn into a nightmare. The thought of this haunted me, and I decided to scratch the book.

Pressure To Share The Information

As I was working on this book, people began to pressure me to put in a section on training and pregnancy. People saw Angela on a TV commercial and on the cover of my books, and they were all saying, "Come on, you've got to put this information out. Your wife looks fantastic!"

But I still thought, no, I'm not going to stick my neck out. Then the pressure really started. I had been working with supermodel Elaine Irwin Mellencamp for a couple of years. She also had two back-to-back pregnancies, and had gotten back into great shape. (And when I say great shape, I mean great shape. She has recently appeared on the cover of *Shape* Magazine and Victoria's Secret catalogs.) With the publicity of Elaine's modeling, people began to really pressure me to put this information out.

I have never changed my mind about publishing Baby Fat. I still don't plan to ever publish it. But I do feel the information I've learned is important to share and would be very beneficial to women who face the challenge of pregnancy.

Our Pregnancy Experiment

Angela trained before, during, and after the first pregnancy. While we are not covering the exact program she used before the pregnancy, it is important to note that it was a well-rounded, general conditioning program similar to the programs found

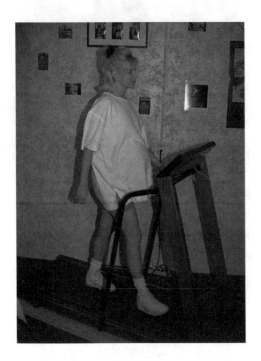

earlier in this book. Angela did not train during or immediately after the second pregnancy.

Both pregnancies were relatively the same—healthy and without complications and neither deliveries were cesarean sections. Obviously, this was not a scientific experiment, but I am confident of the real world applications. Angela ran her business throughout both pregnancies. She wasn't able to stay home, exercise, then sleep all day. She spent most days on her feet, cutting hair in our salon. That makes this even more interesting and applicable in everyday life. This wasn't something she had leisure time to do. This was getting up in the middle of the night, feeding the baby, exercising at 5:30 a.m., arriving at work by 7:30, working on her feet all day until 5:00 p.m., then coming home and taking care of a new born.

It really excited me that our experiment was performed in the laboratory of real life. I have read through piles of research and poured over pages of statistics of experiments based on all kinds of hypothetical situations. But there always seemed to be something missing from these controlled experiments. The missing element was application in the real world. Few people live in a controlled environment and live a laboratory life.

One of the pregnancy and exercise pamphlets that Angela brought home from the doctor's office noted that it had not been clinically proven that exercise benefited pregnancy. I am not sure where the researchers got their information because we found that training before, during, and after pregnancy had significant benefits throughout the entire pregnancy process—both physically and mentally. The benefits included: less weight gain, more energy and endurance, fewer aches and pains (especially in the lower back), less swelling and water retention, higher pain tolerance, fewer "bad food" cravings, more flexibility and mobility, a much quicker recovery, greater self-confidence, better self-image, more mental preparedness for delivery, and fewer mood swings. Our findings shouldn't shock anyone. It's been well proven that partaking in a fitness program adds to the quality of one's life. So, why not during pregnancy?

After the first pregnancy, Angela bounced back quickly. Within 24 hours she felt up to slowly walking on the treadmill. In fact, Angela gave birth around 11 o'clock at night, and the next morning she was able to walk to the car. That was not the case after the second pregnancy when she had not exercised. In fact, lack of exercise made the whole recovery much more difficult. Our experiment showed us the benefits of training during pregnancy. I'm convinced training does have positive effects on pregnancy, and I am also convinced that training is the only way to get back into great shape after the baby is born.

The Program We Developed

We came to the conclusion that it was best to set up the training program to follow the natural pregnancy process. I learned this quickly as we were going through the first pregnancy. This isn't something I thought of in advance or would have been able to learn from research. Most doctors and medical publications will give you a general exercise program and tell you to follow it through your pregnancy until you feel uncomfortable with it. But as most women know, the game changes in each trimester. Just like in any successful training program, making the proper adjustments is the key to success.

First Trimester

As I mentioned, Angela was already following a general training program before she became pregnant the first time. She was training three days a week. Monday she would do weight training for the chest, shoulders, abdominals, legs and then aerobic exercise for 20 minutes, usually treadmill or bike. Wednesdays she would train her biceps, triceps, legs, abs, and then bike for 15 minutes of aerobic exercise at the end. Fridays she would train her back, legs, stomach, and get in 30 minutes of aerobic exercise on the treadmill or bike. That was the program she followed before she became pregnant.

I believe most women can continue to follow their pre-pregnancy training program, but they will need to make adjustments to it. During the first trimester, the most important adjustment is to the length, intensity, and duration of the sessions. This is because there is so much fatigue in the first trimester, more than during any other trimester. We found it necessary to cut back and lighten up each training session. We kept the same program, but we eased up by eliminating sets and reps, lightening weights, and cutting back on the intensity and length of aerobic exercise. Comfort-wise, Angela was able to do all the exercises she had been performing pre-pregnancy, with the exception that I cut all lower abdominal exercises. (The stomach is starting to stretch and expand, and I didn't feel like it made sense to keep training it.)

She followed this program for the first trimester. There were times she was very fatigued, and she would listen to her body and make adjustments. Take your training day to day, and remember to always listen to your body. It is the best coach.

Second Trimester

During the second trimester, we started to make significant changes. Angela still followed the same basic program and trained three days a week, but her stomach was beginning to protrude, and I could see some exercises would soon become uncomfortable. I decided to make changes before that became the case. On Monday she still worked the chest, shoulders, and legs but we made an adjustment on the abdominals—no more abdominal work, upper or lower. Wednesday she trained her biceps, triceps, and legs. Friday she worked her back and legs. Each of the three days she ended her training with aerobic work.

In fact, the amount of aerobic work was another adjustment to the training program. Angela's energy started to pick back up in the second trimester. We began to focus more on cardiovascular work and less on the weights. By this point most women have gained at least 10-15 pounds. The body is bigger, so it's not the time to add any size with weights. We kept the weights light and the reps between 15-25. We also started to eliminate some exercises that were more muscle-mass size building, like the leg press. Instead, Angela started using her body weight to do body squats.

Special Considerations

There are a couple of cautions to be aware of when exercising beyond the first trimester. First is proper back support. The abdominal muscles support the spine, that's one of their functions. This is why many lower back problems can be attributed to weak abdominals. One of the things that happens during pregnancy is that the abdominals loosen and stretch. Because of this and the extra weight of the baby, many pregnant women complain about their backs. When training, make sure your back is always supported so you will avoid back injuries.

Also, it has been recommended by the medical community that women should avoid exercising in the supine position after the first trimester because exercising in this position may be associated with decreased cardiac output in pregnant women. We adjusted all the exercises to avoid lying on the back. Despite these concerns, we can still work the whole body safely with these exercises.

Monday's Training

The best exercise for working the chest muscles is the chest press exercise, normally performed with a barbell or dumbbell while lying in a supine position. With the concern over lying on the back, however, we switched to the **incline dumbbell chest press**, adjusting the bench to a 45-degree angle setting. The second exercise we used for the chest was the **incline dumbbell fly**.

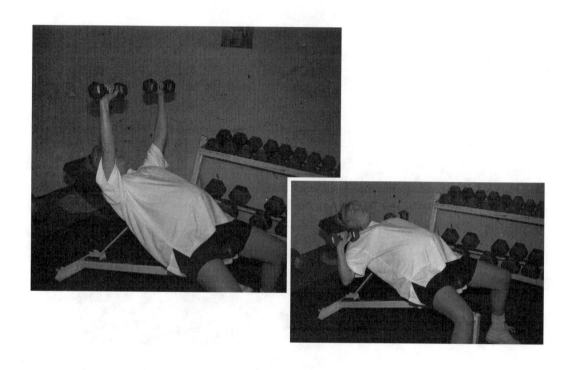

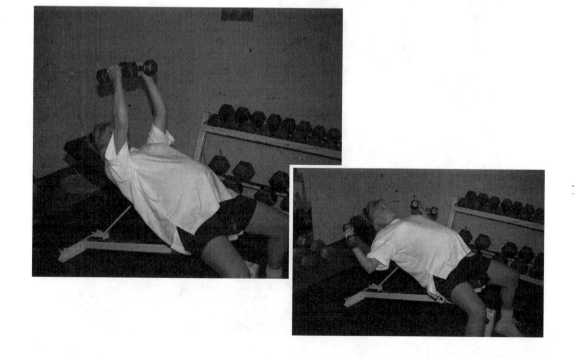

For the shoulders, we used the seated **dumbbell shoulder press**. It's important to note that if you choose to use this exercise, you must use a bench that adjusts to a 90-degree angle to adequately support the back. Pressing movements above the head are sometimes not recommended, but Angela had no problem with the light weights we were using. The second exercise we used for the shoulders was the **seated dumbbell lateral raise**. Both are great exercises for shaping the muscles of the shoulder.

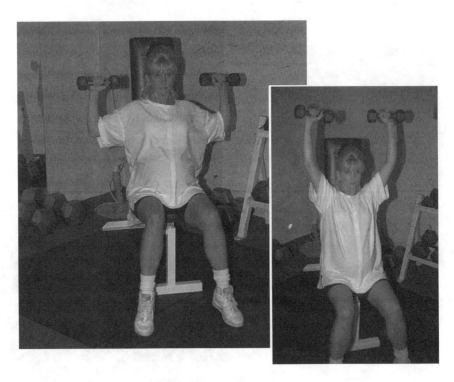

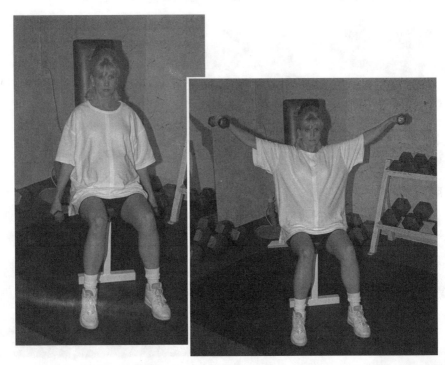

For the legs, the main exercise we used was the **body squat**. As I mentioned earlier, this was a switch from the first trimester where we used the leg press machine. At this point with the protrusion of the lower stomach, I felt using the leg press, which forces your legs down on top of your midsection, was uncomfortable and somewhat unsafe. Angela performed body squats using only her body weight for resistance. The second reason for making this switch was that she did not want to put any size on in the lower body area. I see many women make the mistake of continuing to train with heavy weights throughout their pregnancies, not realizing that the muscles in the lower body naturally increase in size as the pregnancy progresses. This, of course, is caused by the extra weight of the baby. The legs have to accommodate for that extra weight. The baby becomes a sort of permanent weight plate. Every time you climb steps, walk, or get out of a chair, you're lifting the extra pounds. The legs develop more to accommodate for this. Women who continue to train their legs with heavy weights can develop blocky-looking hips, thighs, and calves, which normally isn't the look they are shooting for.

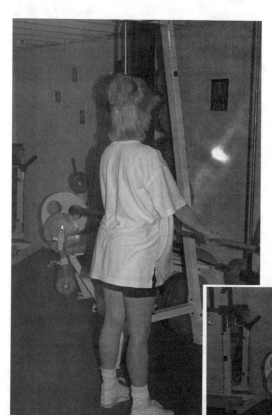

The second exercise we used for the legs was the **leg extension**. This exercise is easy and safe to perform because you're in a back-supported, seated position. It places no pressure on the lower back. Keep in mind we kept the weights light, to avoid putting any extra size on the thighs.

NOTE—One exercise that is used for targeting the back of the thigh is the lying leg curl. This exercise should NOT be used during pregnancy because of the obvious discomfort and potential danger of lying on your stomach. If, however, you have access to a seated curl machine, that is safe to use.

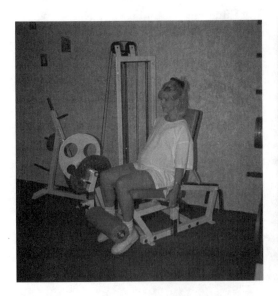
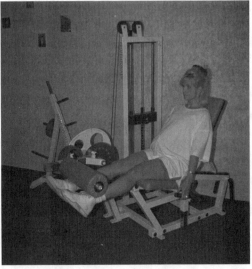

The last exercise for the legs was the **standing calf raise**. This is a great exercise for working the entire calf area. Again, we used only her body weight to avoid adding size to the calf area.

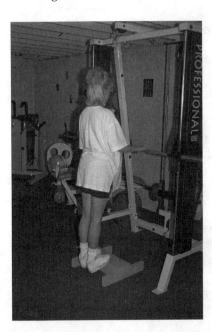
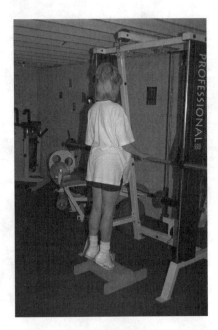

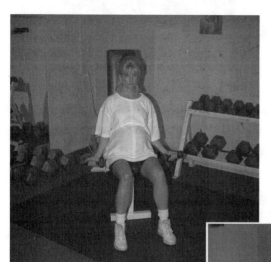

Wednesday's Training

On Wednesdays Angela trained her arms and legs. The first exercise she used was the **seated dumbbell arm curl**. This exercise was performed in a seated position with the bench pad set at a 90-degree angle to support the lower back. In this position the exercise was safe and comfortable to perform.

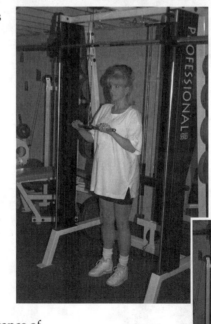

The second exercise for the arms was the **standing tricep cable pushdown**. This exercise is great for working the back of the arms, an area that many of my female clients complain gets soft and flabby during pregnancy.

For the legs she did the same exercises: body squats, leg extensions, and standing calf raises. The only adjustment she made was varying her foot position in the body squat exercise. Sometimes she would take a narrow stance of about 6 inches apart and sometimes she would widen her stance to 8-12 inches. This helps change the emphasis of the exercise and gives the muscles in the area more complete development.

Friday's Training

On Friday Angela worked her back and legs. For the back Angela used the **lat machine pulldown**. This exercise is great for working the muscles of the back, and when performed in a seated position, this exercise is safe and comfortable to use. However, if you are performing this exercise on a commercial lat pulldown machine, you may have to sit backward on the machine because the knee-hold pads may not allow you to sit comfortably.

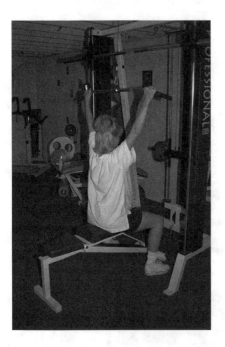 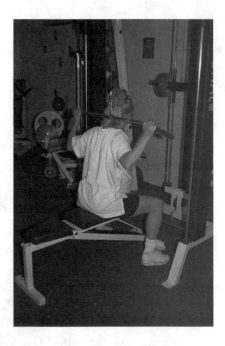

The second exercise for the back was the **bent over one arm dumbbell row**. Another great exercise for working the back muscles, this exercise was comfortable and safe to perform. For legs she repeated the same exercises—body squats, leg extension, standing calf raises.

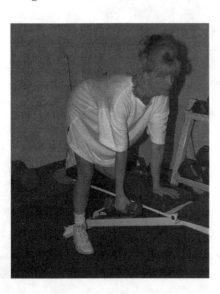 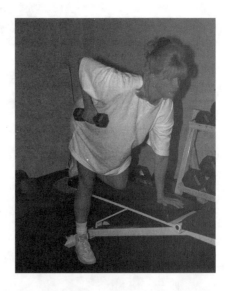

Aerobic Training

Angela ended each training session with aerobic work. She usually did 30 minutes on Monday, 40 minutes on Wednesday, and 25 minutes on Friday. That was up from the first trimester because she now had more energy, was feeling better, and felt like training more. She was also experiencing some water retention and swelling so she wanted to get in more aerobic exercise. We increased her cardiovascular time and cut her weights down, sometimes just to one set.

Its important to note that at no point did she let herself get overheated. She was careful not to overdress or get her heart rate up too high. By wearing a heart monitor, she was able to make the necessary adjustment if she was working too hard. I strongly recommend that you purchase a heart rate monitor to ensure the safety of your workouts.

The treadmill was the only piece of exercise equipment that Angela felt comfortable on after the first trimester. At this point her protruding stomach made the bike and stair climber much too uncomfortable.

Third Trimester

In the third trimester, Angela performed the same exercises as in the second trimester, but she cut back to one set of each exercise keeping the reps around 15. By now she was becoming uncomfortable, not so much in exercising but just with being pregnant in general. We continued to focus on her aerobic work. The weight training was short, usually 15-20 minutes each session. She still felt good staying on the treadmill sometimes up to 60 minutes. She followed that routine up until about two weeks before her due date. I suspect the sessions may have been as psychologically beneficial as they were physically beneficial. By the ninth month, many women are tired of waiting and are tired of being bigger than normal. The mental benefits of training helped Angela through this difficult period.

Two weeks before she delivered, she stopped all training. She was tired, uncomfortable, and didn't feel up to training. She listened to her body and rested up for the big day.

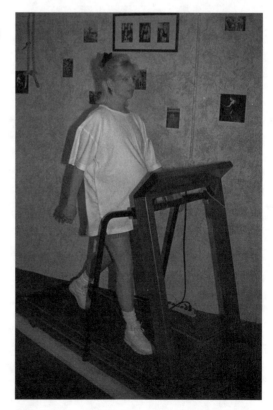

Nutrition and Pregnancy

During her pregnancy, Angela ate 4-5 small meals throughout the day. This worked well to control hunger, prevent cravings, and provide energy. She began and ended each day with supplements in the form of a milkshake to ensure her body was getting all the vital nutrients it needed.

I hesitate to list her exact meal plan because it isn't a meal plan that will work for everyone. One thing about nutrition is that there is not a one-size-fits-all eating plan. We are individuals, but many nutritionists forget this. They come up with a meal plan that works for them and then go about recommending it for everyone on the planet. This is why it is possible for two different people following the same meal plan to get entirely different results. One may lose weight while the other one gets fatter. Nutrition is a very important element in pregnancy. After all, in pregnancy your body becomes a factory—the product it manufactures is a baby and the food you eat is the raw material that helps the baby grow. It is that simple. Pregnancy is NOT a time for dieting—it's a time for sensible eating. Sensible eating means adopting good nutritional habits. Keep this in mind as you develop your nutritional program.

Chapter 17
Training After Pregnancy

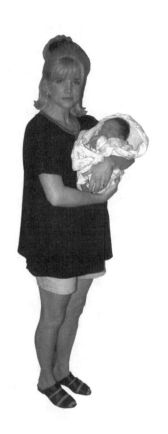

This is probably really frustrating for most women: the baby is born, the pictures have been taken, the hospital has given you a bill, the doctor has dismissed you, and you're wheeled out the door and sent on your way. After my wife's first pregnancy, she asked the nurses at the hospital when she could return to her training program. They gave her a pamphlet that detailed eight floor stretch-type exercises. "You can do these immediately," she was told. "How about real exercise?" she asked. "You can go about your normal exercise routine whenever you feel up to it," was the reply. So much for specifics.

After taking Angela home from the hospital, I began reading through the pamphlet the nurse had given her. I thought, "These exercises are supposed to get her body back in shape?" Looking at my wife's still pregnant-looking body, I knew it would take a lot more than those passive floor exercises. I threw the pamphlet away.

Training is my business. Our livelihood depends on physical conditioning; so there was some pressure in the air. I knew how important getting back in to shape was to Angela. I could tell she was concerned and even a bit doubtful that her body could return to its pre-pregnancy shape. I thought to myself, "I better develop a program that is going to help my wife get back into shape, or things are not going to be good around my house."

The look in Angela's eyes told me that she wanted to start training right away...like as soon as we got home!

I spent the rest of the day thinking about how best to set up her training program and how to safely start on it right away.

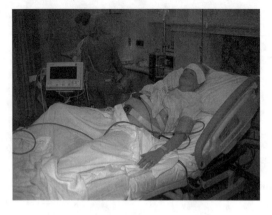

While I have obviously never been pregnant, I have suffered pinched nerves in my lower back. Having a bone deformity coupled with the intense training schedule I follow has sidelined me numerous times with severe lower back injuries. Watching my wife maneuver herself from the car to the couch reminded me of those times. Because of all the nerves centered there, and because this area is the center of all movement, a pinched nerve in the lower back shuts you down! You can't sit up, sleep, put on your socks, go to the bathroom, sneeze, cough, fart, do anything! You can't even lie down comfortably. It's miserable!

The first time that it happened, I went to the hospital. The doctor prescribed pain killers and two weeks of complete bed rest. That turned out to be a form of mental and physical torture. After two days my injury was worse, my brain felt dead, and I was so mentally strained that I was ready to start heavy drinking. Taking matters into my own hands, I developed a training program that I used to quickly recover from injuries like that. Just last year I slipped on a wet side walk while carrying a weight machine. Catching myself, I buckled my knees and pinched a nerve in my lower back. Using my post-injury training program, what normally took weeks to recover from was 80% better in 48 hours.

It dawned on me the quickest and best way to get Angela back into training post-delivery was to train her like I had trained myself after my back injuries. Treat and train her as an injured person; put her through a sort of post-pregnancy rehab program!

Training Angela after her pregnancy taught me that it was best to approach post pregnancy in three phases: phase one—train for recovery, phase two—get back into general condition, and phase three—specific body shaping.

Phase One—Recovery

I call phase one recovery because delivering a baby is traumatic to the body. After having a baby, you're basically an injured person, not unlike an athlete who's had knee surgery or someone who's suffered a back injury. The first priority is to rehabilitate the injury.

With pregnancy you can get a jump on recovery because you know in advance that the delivery (injury) is coming. You can actually start the healing process before you get to the hospital. You may wonder how your body can heal before it is even injured. It can't, but in this case you are expecting the injury and you can get a head start on supplying your body with the nutrients it needs to rebuild and repair itself. The day Angela's water broke, we started increasing her nutrient intake. She

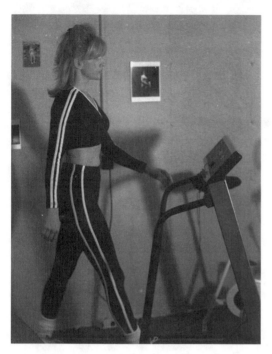

had two or three nutritional shakes over the course of the day. Her first meal after delivering the baby was also a nutrient shake. Loading up on nutrients is intelligent because it provides your body with the building blocks it needs to use to repair itself. Recovery started with nutrients, not exercise.

Two days after delivery, Angela started easy, slow walking on the treadmill. The first couple of weeks she was home, her only exercise was the treadmill, keeping the heart rate down to 50-60% of maximum. This was not strenuous walking, just enough to get the heart rate up a little and get the cobwebs outs. The focus was to get her moving. This is important for recovery because getting the heart rate up gets the blood flowing which flushes nutrients throughout the body and removes waste products and oxygenates the blood. All of this aides recovery. Remember, gentle exercise; you're not running a race!

The first time on the treadmill she only walked about 10 minutes. The second time it jumped to 15 minutes. Because she felt comfortable exercising, Angela's time on the treadmill steadily climbed with each session. Before and after each treadmill session, Angela did some gentle stretches. It is important to stay flexible. There were no weights the first three weeks. She wanted to walk everyday, but I thought it was best to train every other day to give her body more recovery time.

By the end of the third week she was ready to start lifting weights. Some people may need longer than that. Be sure and listen to your body. Don't try to push ahead before you are ready. Keep this warning in mind: If you push too hard too fast, you're going to have problems.

What's important to remember in phase one of post-pregnancy training is to continually flood the system with nutrients, use moderate cardiovascular exercise to help speed recovery, and gently stretch to keep the muscles limber and flexible.

Phase Two—General Conditioning

As with any injury, the lack of activity normally causes muscle atrophy, strength loss, body fat gain, and a decline in aerobic fitness. When you stop exercising, the body rapidly starts to lose conditioning.

This was the case with Angela. As I mentioned in Chapter Sixteen, she had stopped exercising two weeks before delivery. Add in the three weeks that she spent in phase one recovery exercise, and she had not strenuously exercised for five weeks. Her body had lost quite a bit of tone and shape, and she had accumulated some unwanted body fat from the pregnancy.

Angela was eager to start working with light weights. The back and stomach muscles still need to be supported, so we used the same exercises we did in the second trimester. Angela started those with one set each of 15 reps, followed by about 10 minutes of cardiovascular work. These were the exercises we used:

Incline Dumbbell Press

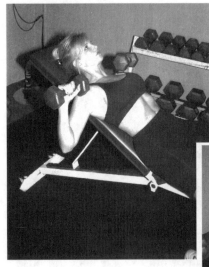
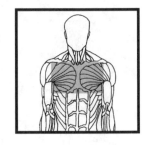
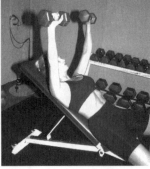

Incline Dumbbell Fly

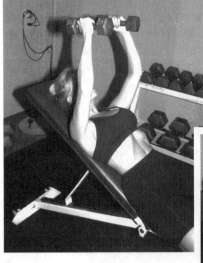
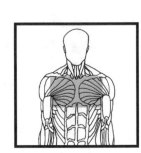
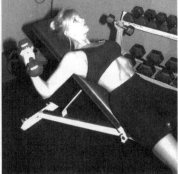

Lat Machine Pulldown

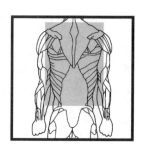

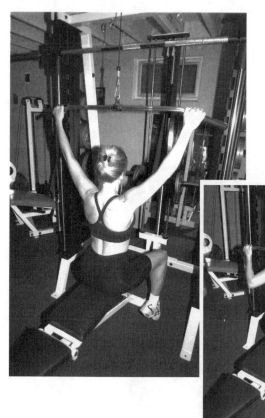

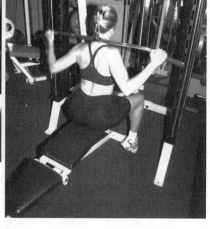

Bent Over One Arm Dumbbell Row

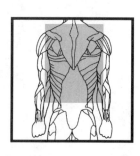

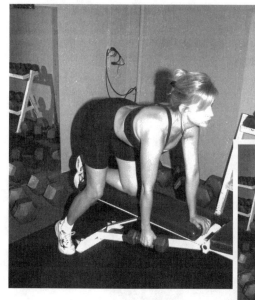

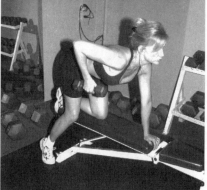

Seated Dumbbell Press

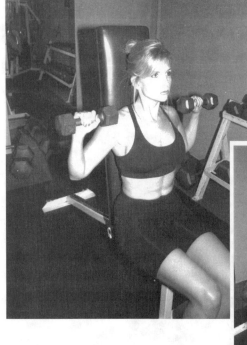
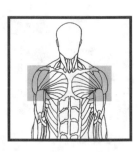
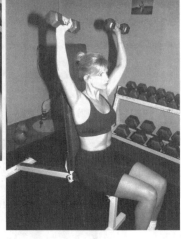

Seated Dumbbell Lateral Raise

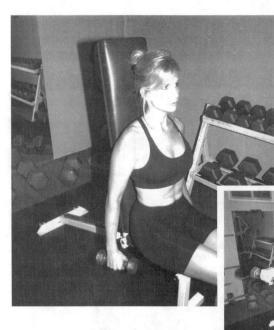
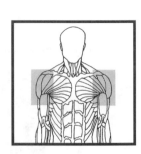

Seated Dumbbell Arm Curl

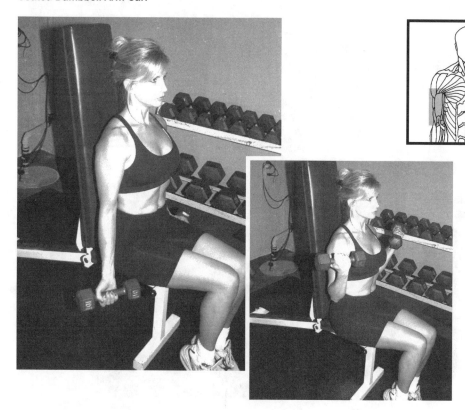

Tricep Cable Pushdown

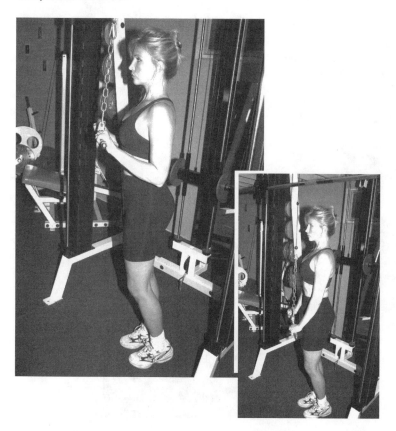

Body Squat

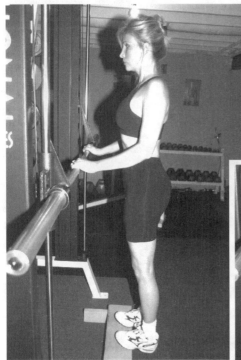
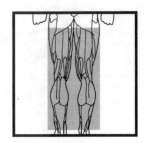
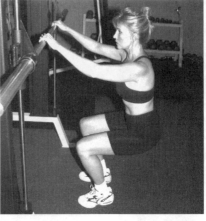

Leg Extension

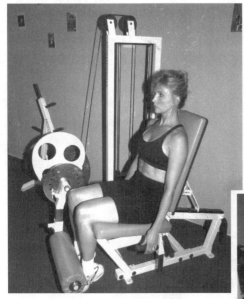
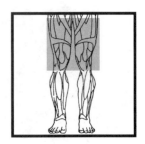
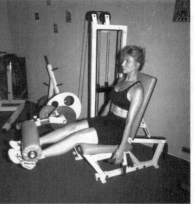

Standing Calf Raise

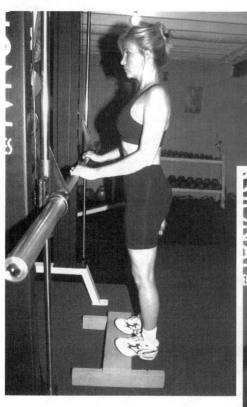
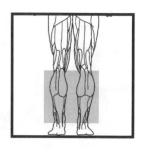
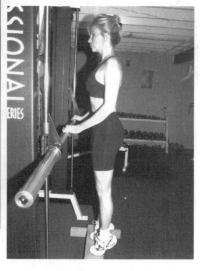

Crunch

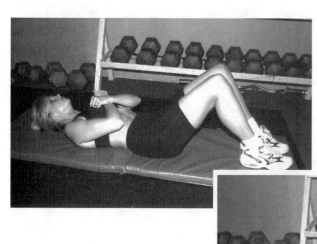
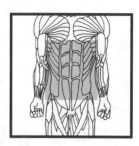

Incline Bench Knee-ups

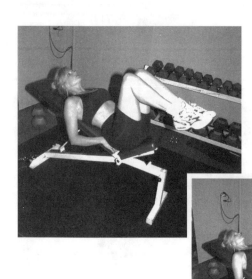
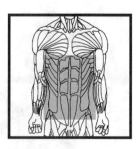

Hyperextension

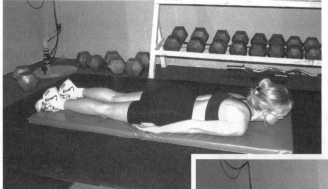
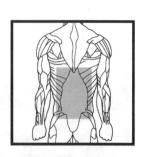
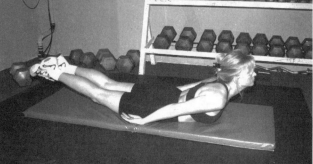

I was amazed at the progress Angela made from one day to the next. By her third week in phase two, she was ready to really get into the weights. The timing on that is really a personal decision. Don't push too soon. For two more weeks she increased the sets and reps. Angela spent about six weeks in phase two getting her body back into general condition. Her strength had returned and her cardiovascular system was back in shape so she could easily do 30 to 40 minutes keeping her heart rate in the 75-80% target range.

Phase Three—Body Shaping

When Angela felt like she was back into good general condition, she was ready to begin more advanced training and do some specific body shaping. After the pregnancy she wanted some extra work on the backs of her arms, her thighs, and lower stomach. Using the body-specific exercises in Section Two, we customized her program and added extra exercises for her trouble spots.

Rest assured you can get your body back to its pre-pregnancy shape. It can be even better—I've seen it proven! Having a baby does not mean you have to lose your figure. You can get back in shape, but it takes some work and good effort. If you approach it intelligently, it's not as challenging as you might think. Just realize that exercise and nutrition are going to be a part of it. I find that if a woman has trained before and during pregnancy, she can be back into great shape in a couple of months.

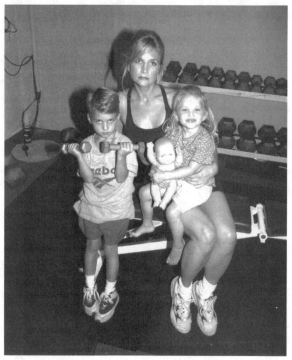

Keys to Know

These are some things that will help you with your post-pregnancy program. Make exercise a priority. With all the pressure of parenthood, you may be tempted to make excuses for not exercising. The benefits of exercising after pregnancy are not just physical. Exercise can help with postpartum depression. You're taking on a new, demanding challenge. The better you feel about yourself, the better you will feel about your ability to cope. Again, make exercise a priority.

Also, don't expect baby to conform to your schedule. Your best bet is to conform to his, and the only way to do this is by being flexible. I recommend getting dumbbells, a weight bench, and a treadmill to keep in your home. That way you have the freedom to get in a workout while the baby is napping, instead of trying to find a sitter while you run to the gym. Enjoy the baby when he is awake, and get in a workout while he is asleep! Another great piece of equipment to get is an electric baby swing. With it, you don't have to wait for the baby to go to sleep.

The program I outlined in this chapter worked for my family. Listen to your body and your doctor when planning your own post-pregnancy training program.

Chapter 18
Figure Firming For Women

Although both men, women, boys, and girls can train pretty much the same way—that is, they can perform the same weight training and aerobic exercises and reap many of the same results—I found through my experience of training females that they can benefit with some special twists to their training program.

The current "vogue" look of the models with their sunken cheeks and toneless arms and legs is not only unattractive but unhealthy. A well-toned, shapely, energetic body is by far much more attractive... and healthy.

I am somewhat concerned with women when it comes to diet and exercise. A recent survey conducted by *Shape* magazine surveyed girls ages 11-17 on their body image, exercise, and eating habits. The results were scary: many of the survey participants had serious eating disorders and constantly compared themselves to classmates with so-called "perfect bodies"—the ones researchers feared had the more serious eating disorders.

Excessive weight gain and loss of control of body shape can play havoc to your self-image. We all should strive to put our best foot forward, and that includes our physical appearances. An exercise program consisting of weight training, aerobic conditioning, and good nutritional practices is the best way to improve your appearance.

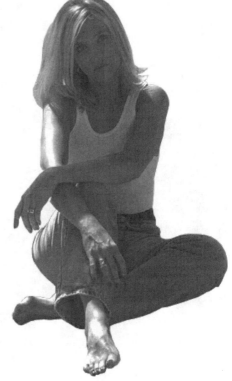

A Great Way To Shape Up The Female Body

Generally women are worried most about controlling body fat, so "diet" is often first the course of action. And what usually follows is a host of problems from eating disorders, to damaging weight loss, depression, and loss of energy and drive. Then follows a rebound of body fat gain. This scenario becomes a never-ending cycle as every new year brings a new miracle weight loss program, product, or pill.

The Answer

The muscles in the body give it its shape and contour. The best way to add shape, symmetry, and tone is through a good weight training program. The other side of the coin is to eliminate body fat. This is best achieved when adding aerobic training.

Figure Firming Program

Figure firming guides you though a routine designed to concentrate on the areas of concern, including hips, thighs, upper arms, and abs. The end result will be a firmer, more proportionate shapely figure. The goals are to lose body fat, develop symmetry and proportion, increase muscle tone, and enhance shape.

Figure Firming Routine

Monday—chest, triceps, abs, aerobic training

Tuesday—legs, abs, fat burning

Wednesday—back, biceps, abs, aerobic training

Thursday—shoulders, abs, fat burning

Friday—legs, abs, aerobic training

Monday—Smith Machine Chest Press

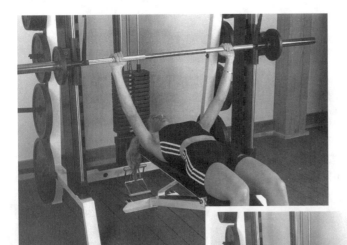
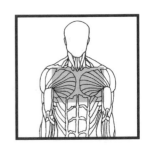

Incline Dumbbell Flys

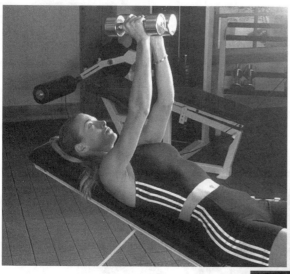
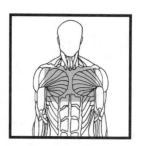
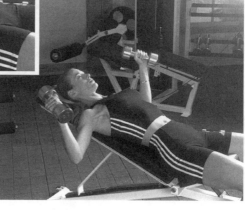

Tricep Cable Pushdown

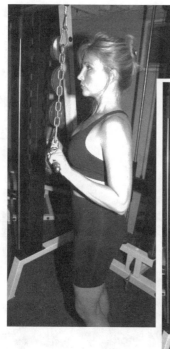
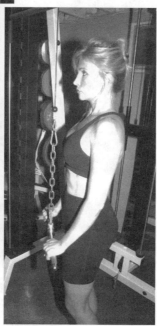
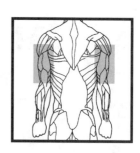

Bench Dip

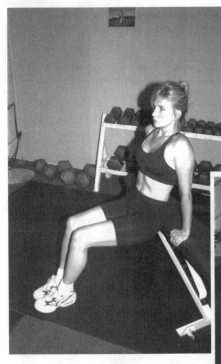
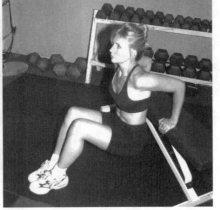
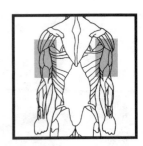

Crunch

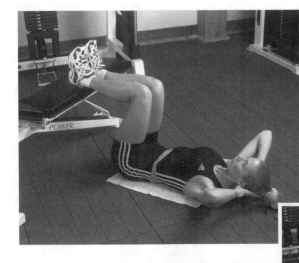
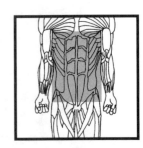

Incline Seated Leg Raise

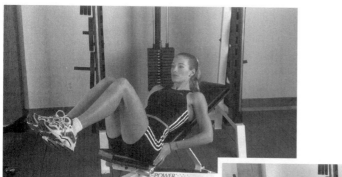
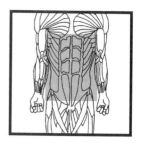
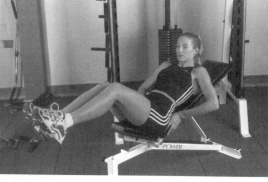

Tuesday—Smith Machine Squat

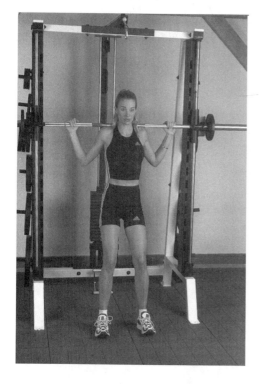
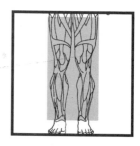
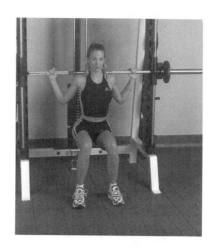

Smith Machine Lunge

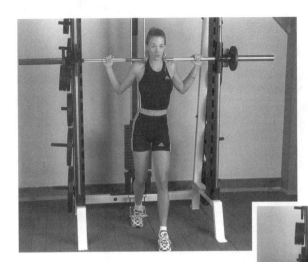
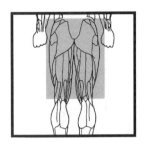

Leg Extension

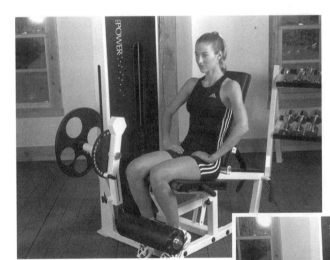
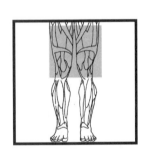

Leg Curl

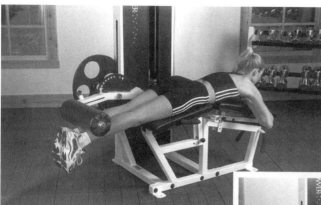
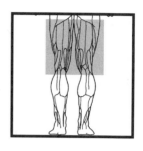
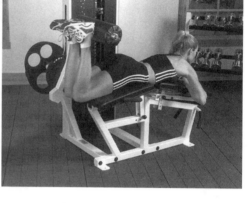

Smith Machine Standing Calf Raise

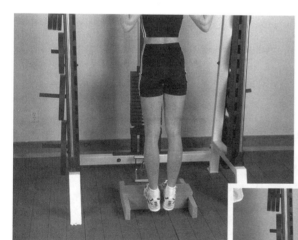
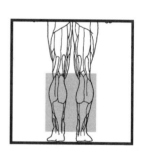

Partial Incline Sit-up

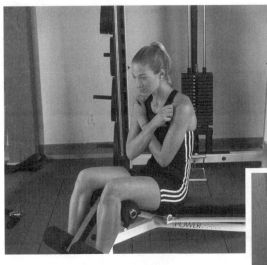
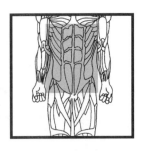
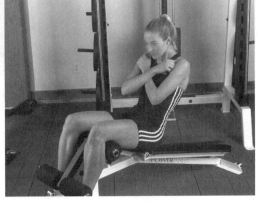

Seated Leg Raise

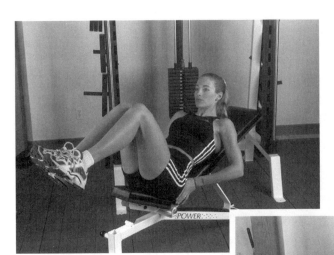
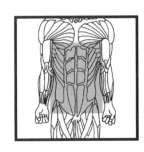

Wednesday—Lat Pulldown

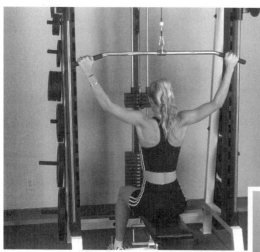
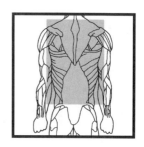
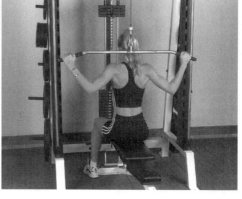

Low Pulley Cable Row

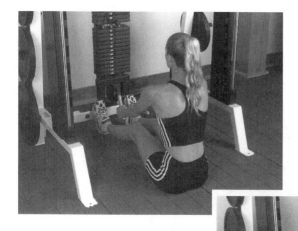
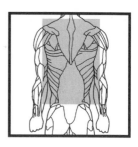

Dumbbell Seated Arm Curl

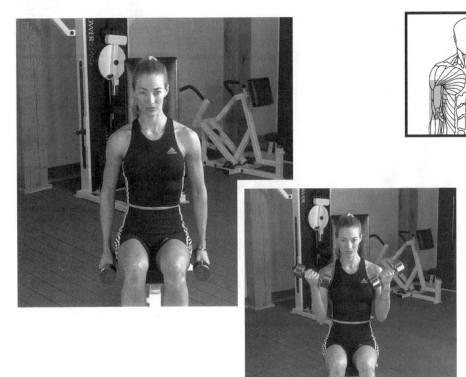

Reverse Crunch

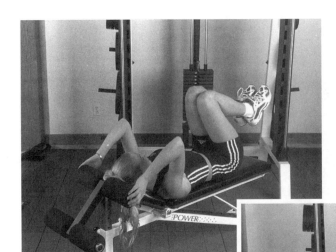

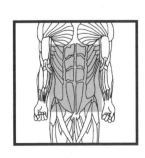

Incline Seated Leg Raise

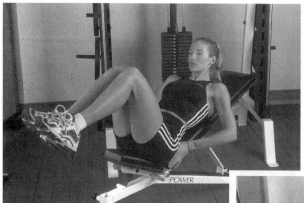
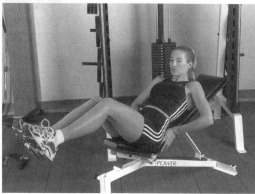

Friday—Smith Machine Shoulder Press (front of neck)

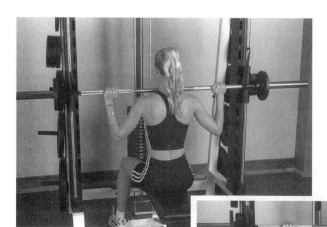
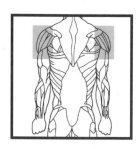

Barbell Upright Row

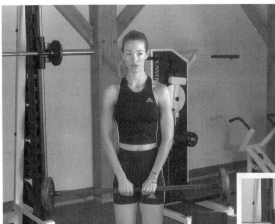
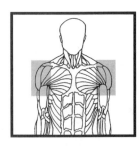
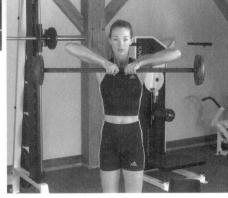

Dumbbell One Arm Front Raise

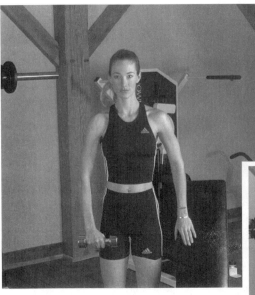
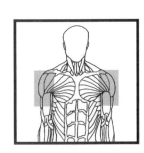
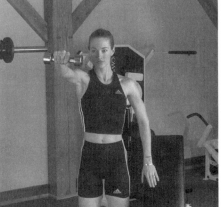

Partial Incline Sit-up

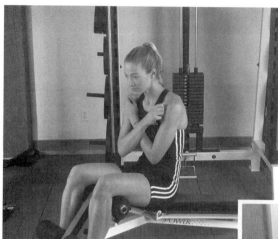
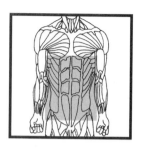
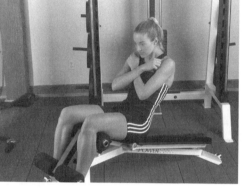

Seated Leg Raise

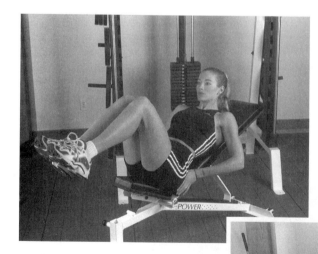
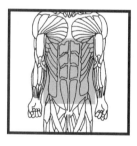

Firday—Smith Machine Squat

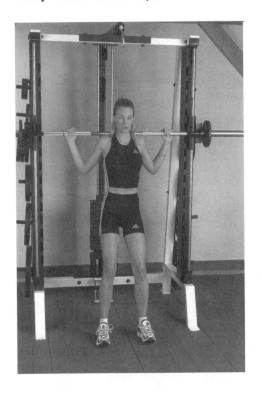
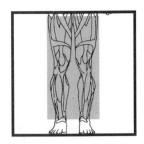
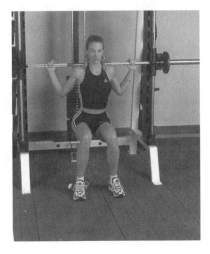

Outter Thigh (repeat opposite side)

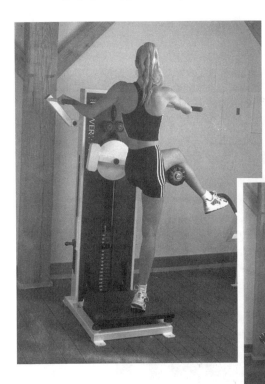
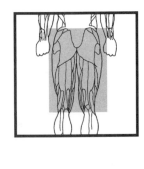

Inner Thigh (repeat with opposite leg)

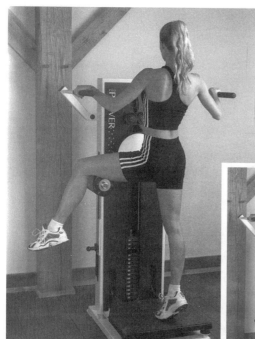
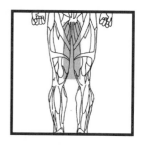
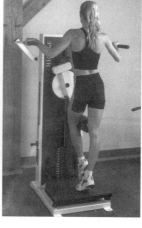

Glute and Hamstring (repeat with opposite leg)

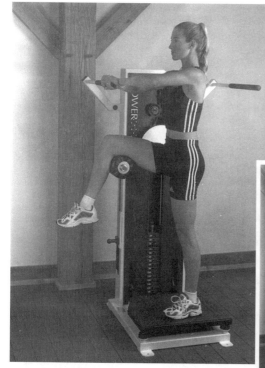
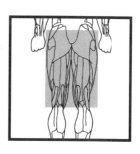
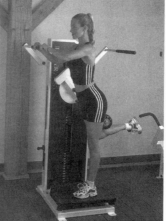

Smith Machine Standing Calf Raise

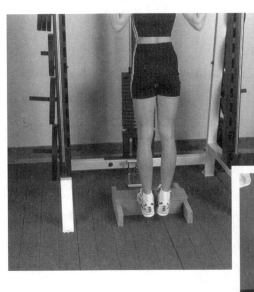
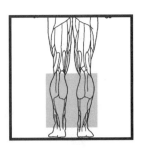
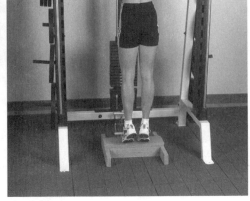

Crunch

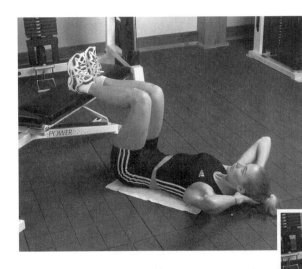
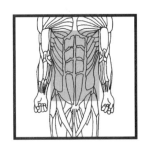

Incline Seated Leg Raise

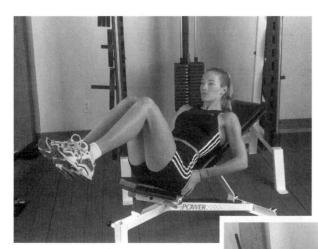
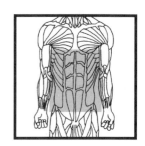

Poundages And Weight

All Upper Body Exercises
Increase weight 5-10 lbs. per set

Lower Body Exercises—Leg Press, Squat, Calf Raise
Increase weight 10-20 lbs. per set

Leg Extension and Leg Curl
Increase weight 5-10 lbs. per set

Nonweight Assisted Exercises—Abdominals, Hyperextensions
Exercise to failure

Sets and Reps

Upper Body Exercises
Between 12-15 reps per set

Lower Body Exercises
Between 15-25 reps per set

Number of sets per exercise
2-3

Rest Between Sets
1-2 minutes

Aerobic Training

Monday after weights
Jog, treadmill, stationary bike, or row, etc.
20 minutes with heart rate in the 75% range

Tuesday after weights
Jog, treadmill, stationary bike, or row, etc.
35 minutes with heart rate in the 65% range

Wednesday after weights
Jog, treadmill, stationary bike or row, etc.
45 minutes with heart rate in the 55% range

Thursday after weights
Jog, treadmill, stationary bike or row, etc.
15 minutes with heart rate in the 75% range

Friday after weights
Jog, treadmill, stationary bike or row, etc.
30 minutes with heart rate in the 60% range

Stretching
Full body stretch after all weight training and aerobic workouts. (See Chapter Nine for key body stretches.)

Chapter 19
Shaping Up Without Weights

Training with weights is the best way to shape your body, however, I realize sometimes weights just are an impossibility.

There are also times when people don't have access to training facilities or can't fit the time to go to the gym into their schedules, but they still want to exercise and stay fit. I'm often asked how do you stay in shape when you're a remote country with no available weight training equipment? Or what about when you're traveling? There are times when you just can't use weights. What do you do during those times?

This chapter contains exercises that can be used when you can't or won't use weights. Keep in mind that these aren't the same as weight training exercises. They're not as good, but they're better than nothing. They're effective enough to maintain shape.

The exercises listed here are my non-weight training program. I've used them in hotels, I've used them in a field in Honduras, I've used them on the side of a mountain in Virgin Gorda, British Virgin Islands. They are effective, and I've relied on them when necessary. I've also used them with young teenagers who were physically not mature enough to handle weights and with adults as entry level into training. They're also good for time crunches or sometimes when you just need a change.

Push-ups

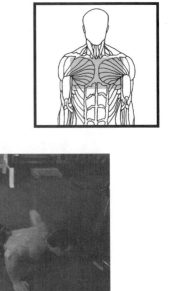

Chair Dip

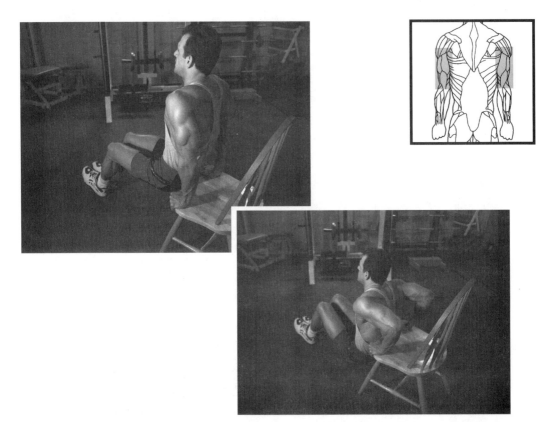

Body squats

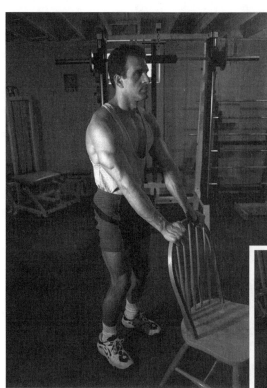
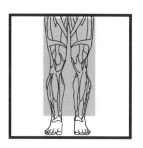
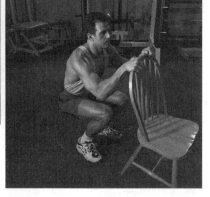

Crunches

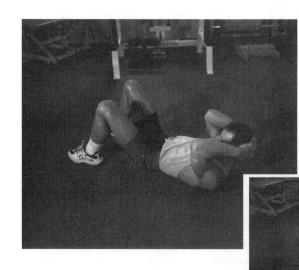
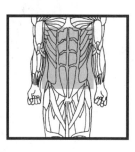

Knee-ups

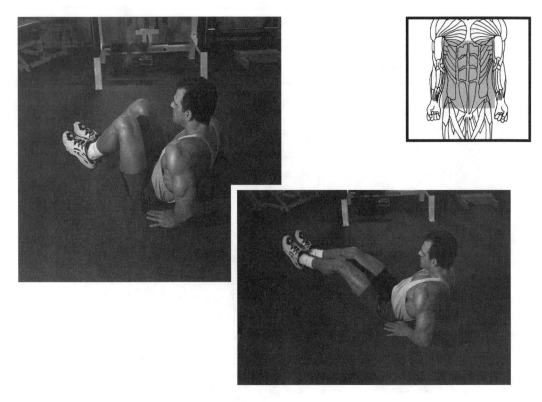

Alternate Crunches

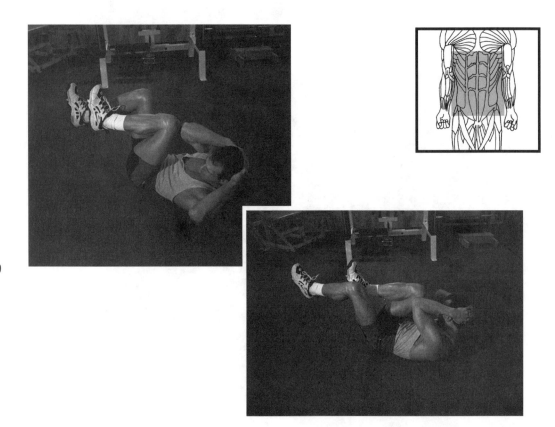

Hyperextensions

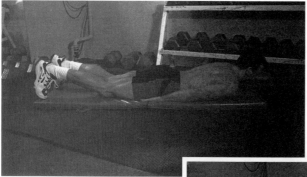
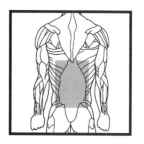
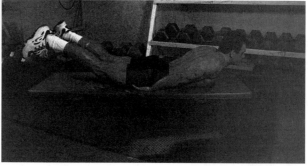

Days
Monday, Wednesday, Friday

Sets and Reps
beginners, 1 set each
intermediate, 2 sets each
advanced, 3 sets each

The number that you do is not important. What is important is that you complete as many as you can with good form. The numbers will always vary because everybody's different. It is better to complete three good push-ups than ten with poor form.

Follow-up with aerobic exercise according to your goals.

Chapter 20
The "I Just Don't Feel Like Training Today" Solution

It happens to everyone—even the most dedicated of athletes. There are times when you just do not feel like training. The very last thing you want to do is get on that treadmill or pick up those dumbbells. Your mind is a million miles away, you have a pile of papers on your desk, your brain is fried, and your body wants a nap. You don't have one drop of energy to get yourself into the gym.

I have been training for over 20 years, and you can bet that there have been many times when I have found myself in this position. I, too, have said to myself, "I just don't feel like training today." But what should you do? Take the day off? Skip your training? That might not be the best answer. You may be experiencing burn out. This is a common problem with a simple solution.

Burn out often stems from falling into a training rut. It is usually a sign that a change is needed. This is not the time to rely on will power to get through the next workout. Forcing yourself through the same old workout can make you more fatigued and wreck your motivation.

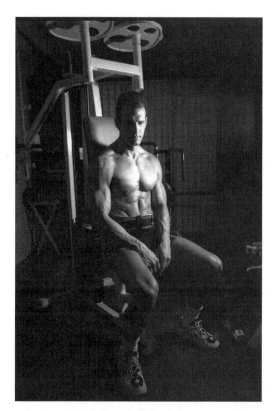

The best prescription for burn out is a change in routine. By making a change you stimulate and regenerate your motivation to get back to your normal training program. The key isn't how you change the routine, but that you change it and get out of your rut. Since a majority of my training centers around weights, when I am burnt I will do only aerobic exercise. I stay out of the gym for a couple of days. Instead, I will go for a 20 minute jog, stretch, and that is it! I mix it up—run outside in the winter, or on the treadmill in the summer—the opposite of what I normally do. I might run hills or stadium steps, put on a heart monitor and go for a bike ride, jog the track at the high school—anything that is different from my normal routine!

If you are burned out on cardio work, you might try going into the weight room and doing one set of every exercise you can think of. I have used this many times with my clients, and they always enjoy the change.

Not only will this satisfy your training obligation, but it will help you avoid any guilt that normally comes from skipping training completely. It always freshens up my mind and body, leaving me eager to get back to my regular training programs.

The key to making it through these times is to "break the pattern," stimulate your body and mind with a new activity or make a normal activity different by altering it in some way. Of course, the best way to treat burn out is to avoid it in the first place. Update your training program and shake things up from time to time. Keep your sessions interesting and you will experience fewer of those "I-just-don't-feel-like-training" days.

Chapter 21
Training "Under The Weather"

I am often asked how people should handle training when they are feeling under the weather—not with a serious illness, but just with a common cold or the flu.

Most people believe there isn't much to be done but bed rest. I have faced this dilemma many times over the course of my training career. I've learned that avoiding the gym did not make me feel better or help me recover more quickly. For me bed rest was always a form of mental and physical torture. As a matter of fact, the few times I tried it, I felt worse and did not get better any faster than the times I continued training through it.

Taking a week off from training because of the sniffles is not something that many people want to do. After years of hard work, the last thing I want to do is start over every time I get sick. Interruptions in a training program always make it hard to restart. Once the training habit is broken, it becomes much more challenging to get going again. We have all seen people blazing along with their training only to get sidelined with a cold and never make it back into the gym.

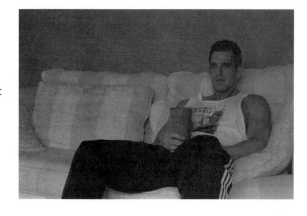

I have found if done properly, exercising when under the weather can help speed recovery and get you back on your feet more quickly without any major set backs in your conditioning. The trick, of course, is to do just the right amount of activity, which is something you will have to experiment and learn for yourself.

Listen to your body. Don't try to prove how tough you are by "sweating it out." If you push yourself and try to do too much too soon, you will run yourself down and delay recovery. You could make yourself even sicker—just the opposite of what you are trying to do!

When I am sick with the flu, I like to focus mostly on aerobic exercise because its less stressful. Also because I feel like it helps pump the poison out. When you increase your heart rate, your heart pumps fresh blood through the body, bringing in fresh nutrients and removing waste products. During bouts with the flus, colds, and allergies, I usually just cut the duration and lower the intensity of my training sessions by eliminating sets and reps. I still stick with my normal routine and schedule for the most part. I do, however, stay on the cautious side, always keeping in mind not to overdo it.

When you are sick, nobody is really going to be able to answer the question, "Should I train today?" except you. It will take some experimentation and involvement on your part, but once you learn how to train when you're under the weather, you will never have your training program sidelined by the sniffles again.

The following are some under-the-weather training guidelines. You will find them helpful the next time you're not feeling so well:

♦ Never train with a fever. This can cause dehydration and always makes you worse.

♦ Cut all weight training exercises down to one set. Reduce poundages 20-40% and fully catch your breath between sets. Avoid using heavy or maximum weights.

♦ Lower the intensity of aerobic exercise (keep heart rate in the 60-65% range) and cut the workout time down by half.

♦ Don't try to sweat it out. Avoid overheating, saunas, steam, and whirlpools

♦ Get your rest—take a nap, prop your feet up, go to bed early, sleep in an extra hour if possible

♦ Increase your supplement intake. Flood your system with nutrients it needs to recover and get better.

♦ If you are too sick to train, try some light stretching or go for a walk.

Part Two

More Great Exercises For Shaping Up

This section contains more of my favorite training exercises for body parts. In this section I have included a variety of exercises that you can incorporate into your training program to help you zero in on those challenge areas. Or you can substitute these exercises into your program to keep it challenging and fresh. This section contains chapters that outline the specific exercises that shape and develop the chest, back, shoulders, arms, abdominals, legs, and hips and thighs. These exercises are great for adding variety and giving your body that little extra attention that it may need to get into great shape.

Chapter 22
More Great Exercises For The Chest

Chest Anatomy

The pectoral consists of two parts—the clavicular (upper) portion and the sternal (lower) portion. The upper part is attached to the clavicle (collarbone). Along the mid body line, it attaches to the sternum (breastbone) and to the cartilage of several ribs. The largest mass of the pectoral starts at the upper arm bone (humerus), fastened at a point under and just above where the deltoids attach to the humerus. The pectorals spread out like a fan and cover the rib cage like plates. Attached to the rib cage in the center and across to the shoulder, this muscle lets you perform such motions as pitching a ball underhanded, doing a wide arm bench press, or twisting a cap off a bottle.

Training The Chest

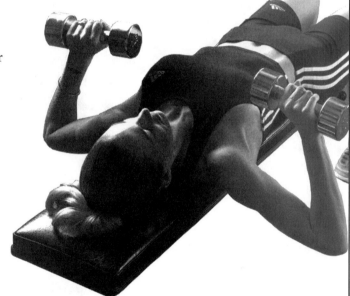

The two basic exercises for the chest are presses (you press the weight away from the chest) and flys (you draw your extended arms together across the chest in a hugging motion). The chest exercises I have listed are designed to help you achieve the most complete development. To completely develop the back, you need to consider how each of the important back muscles function so that you include exercises that work the entire back region. Complete development means developing the inside, outside, upper and lower areas of the pectoral.

Upper Chest Exercises

Incline Barbell Press

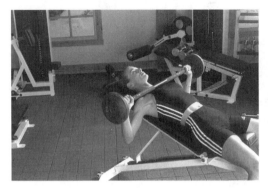
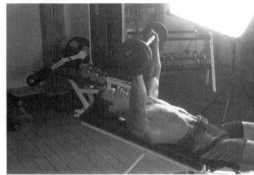

60 Degree High Incline Dumbbell Fly

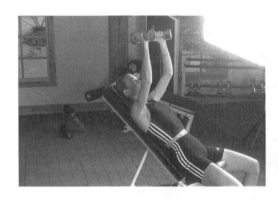
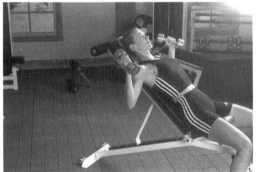

Lower Chest Exercises

Decline Bench Barbell Press

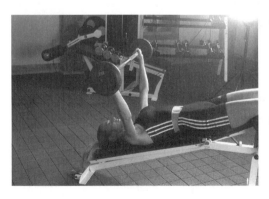
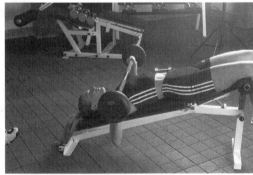

Decline Bench Cable Fly

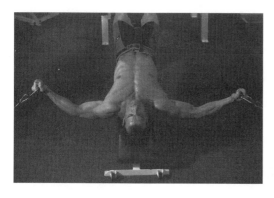 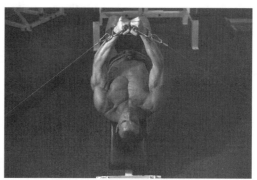

Inner Chest Exercises

Cable Crossover

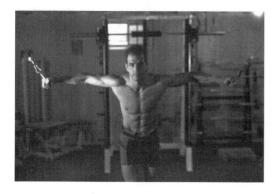 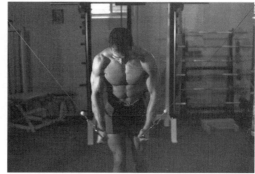

Palms Facing Dumbbell Press

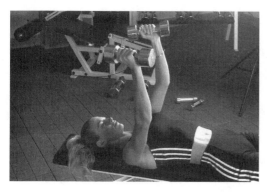 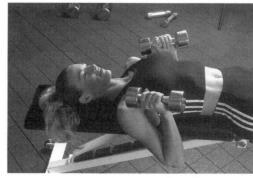

Outer Chest Exercises

Smith Machine Incline Press (wide grip)

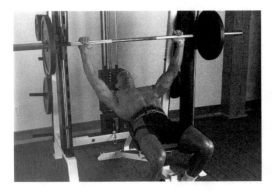 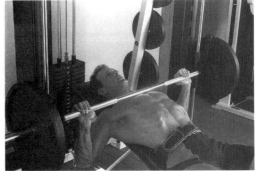

Push-up (wide hand placement)

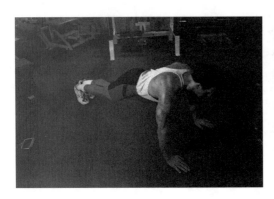 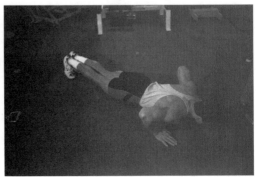

Chapter 23
More Great Exercises For The Back

Back Anatomy

The flat triangular muscle that extends out and down from the neck and down between the shoulder blades is the trapezius. The trapezius' primary function is to raise the shoulder girdle. The latissimus dorsi (lats) are the large triangular muscles that extend from under the shoulders down to the small of the back on both sides. Their primary function is to pull the shoulders downward. The spinal erectors, composed of several muscles in the lower back that guard the nerve channels, work to hold the spine erect, straighten the spine from a position with torso flexed completely forward, and help to arch the lower and middle back.

Training The Back

The key to fully developing the back muscles is to isolate the six areas of the back. The back consists of a number of complex and interrelated muscles that do not develop at the same rate; therefore, you should keep this in mind and choose exercises that work each individual part of the back.

Special note: Save lower back exercises until the end of the workout. The lower back muscles are the slowest muscles in the body to recuperate from heavy exercise. Sometimes it may require up to a week for recovery. Therefore, you should perform power exercises, such as deadlifts, using heavy weights, only once a week. However, you may perform non-power exercises, such as hyperextensions, more frequently.

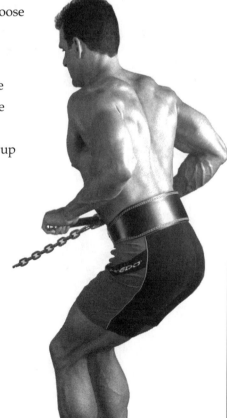

Outer Back Exercises

Standing Narrow Reverse Grip Low Pulley Rows

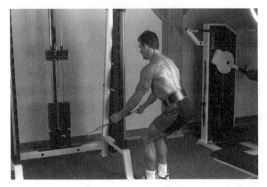
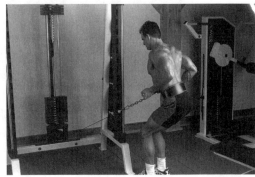

One Arm Low Pulley Rows

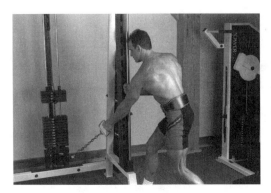
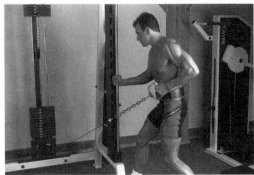

Upper Back Exercises

Smith Machine Reverse Upright Row

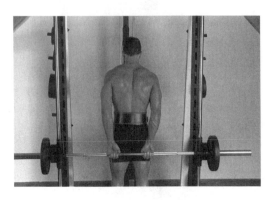
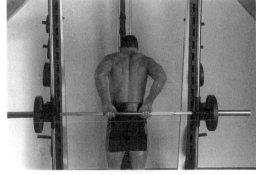

Dumbbell Reverse Upright Row

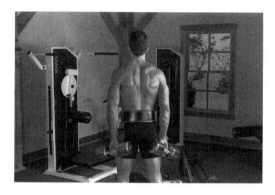
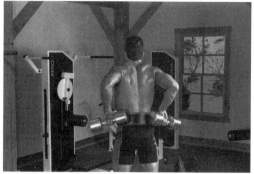

Lat Width Exercises

Wide Grip Pulldowns (front of the neck)

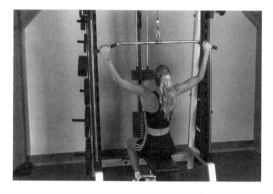
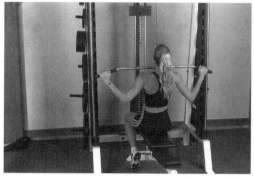

Lower Lat Exercises

Close Grip Pulldowns

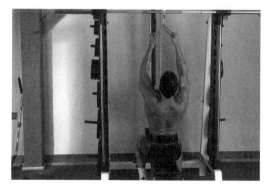
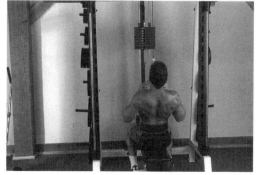

Middle Back Exercises

Stiff Arm Pulldowns

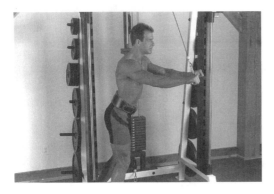 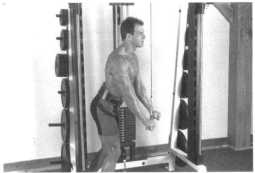

Lower Back Exercises

Low PulleyBack Extension

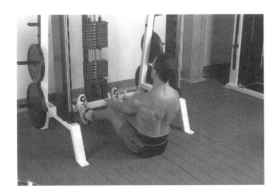 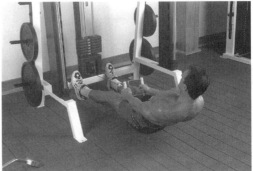

Smith Machine Partial Deadlifts

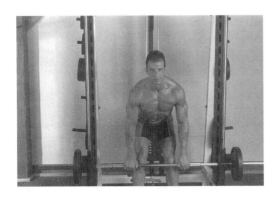 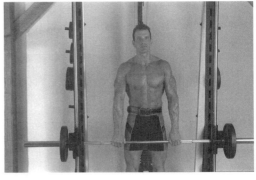

Chapter 24
More Great Exercises For The Shoulders

The deltoids enable your arm to move in a 360 degree circle, and that means there are many angles from which to train your shoulders in order to bring out their full shape and development.

Shoulder Anatomy

The deltoids are versatile muscles that move the arm forward, backward, to the side, up and around. The deltoids have three distinct lobes of muscle called "heads" that enable this movement: the anterior head (the muscle in the front), the medial head (the muscle on the side), and the posterior head (the muscle in the rear).

The two basic exercises for training the deltoids are presses and lateral raises. Shoulder presses begin with arms bent and the weight held about shoulder height. You then lift a barbell or dumbbells straight overhead. You may also perform this exercise on a machine. You can direct the stress to different deltoid heads by doing different kinds of presses—to the front or back.

Laterals involve lifting your extended arm upward in a wide arc. In order to work all three heads, you need to do laterals to the front, to the side and to the rear. When you do laterals, you completely isolate the various heads of the deltoids.

Training The Deltoids

Overall shoulder development means working towards symmetrical development between the three deltoid muscles: the anterior, medial and posterior (front, side and rear). When setting up your shoulder routine, select exercises that stress each of the three areas.

It is very easy to overtrain the shoulders, so be very cautious to limit the number and frequency of shoulder exercises.

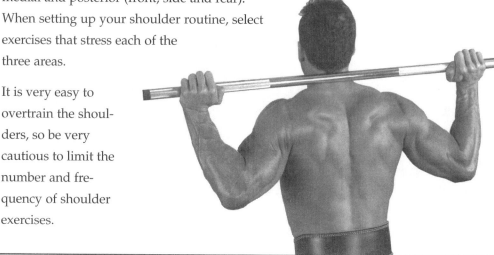

Front Deltoid Exercises (anterior)

Standing Dumbbell One Arm Front Raise

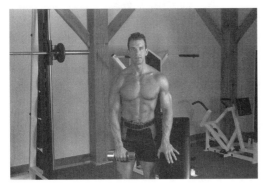
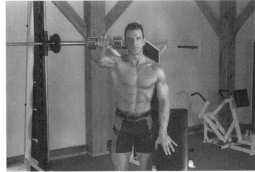

Plate Front Raise

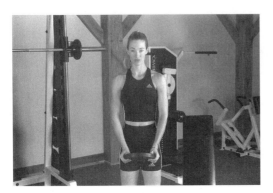
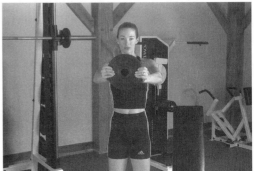

Low Pulley One Arm Front Raise

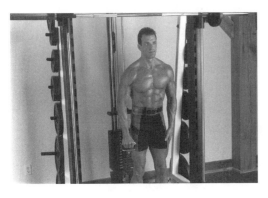
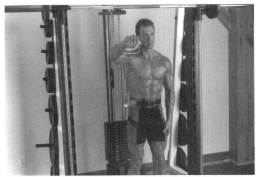

Low Pulley Front Raise

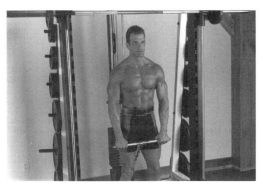
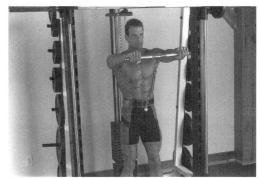

Middle Deltoid Exercises (medial)

High Incline Dumbbell Lateral Raise

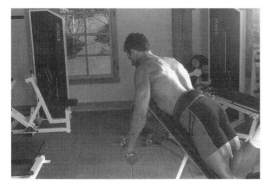
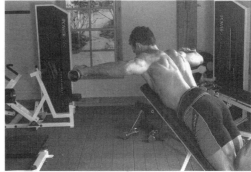

Low Pulley One Arm Lateral Raise

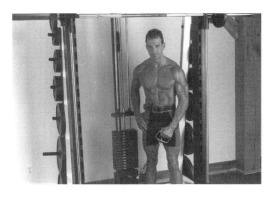
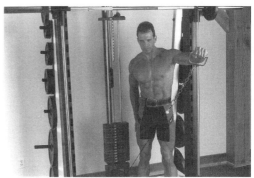

Narrow Grip Upright Row

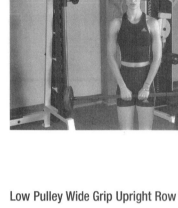
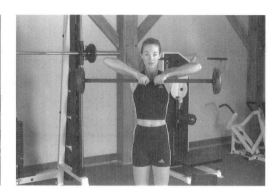

Low Pulley Wide Grip Upright Row

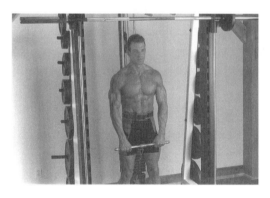
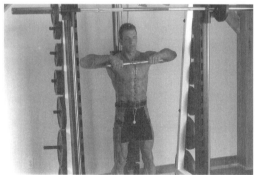

Rear Deltoid Exercises (posterior)

Seated Bent Forward Dumbbell Rear Lateral Raise

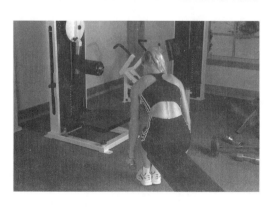
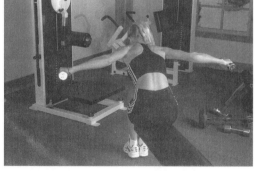

Standing Bent Forward Rear Lateral Dumbbell Raise

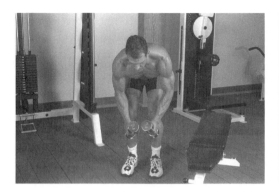
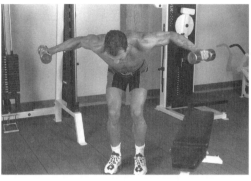

Chapter 25
More Great Exercises For The Biceps

Good arm development is important for both men and women. Achieving good arm development means developing a balance between the biceps, triceps, and forearms.

You can approach arm training in several ways. You can train the whole arm in one workout by either finishing each muscle group before going on to the next or by alternating sets for the biceps and triceps, thus working both sides of the arm at the same time. Or you can break up your training so that you train triceps one day, biceps the next and forearms another day. As with other body parts, the best development will come when you employ a variety of exercises and training techniques.

Anatomy of the Biceps
The biceps (biceps brachii) is a two-headed muscle with its point of origin under the deltoid and its point of insertion below the elbow. There are two muscle groups located at the front of the upper arm that contract to flex the arm fully from a straight position. The smallest of these muscles is called the brachialis, a thin band of muscle between the biceps and triceps. The brachialis muscle runs only about halfway up the humerus bone above the elbow.

The biceps are much larger in mass than the brachialis muscles and are the primary muscle group responsible for bending the arm. With an origin near the shoulder joint and insertions on the forearm bones, the biceps can contract to fully bend the arm from a straight position. The secondary function of the biceps is to supinate (twist) the hand. The biceps make up about 35 percent of the arm mass.

Training the Biceps
People who relate bulging biceps with being totally in shape are wrong. Biceps size and mass are important for defining a well developed biceps muscle; however, shape, definition and complete development are more important than pure size. The barbell curl is the fundamental exercise for developing the biceps.

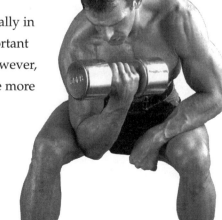

Using a variety of movements to work each of the five areas will give your biceps the best development.

Overall Mass Of Bicep Exercises

Low Pulley Arm Curl

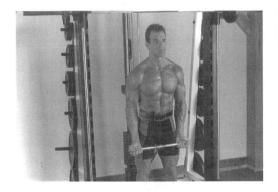
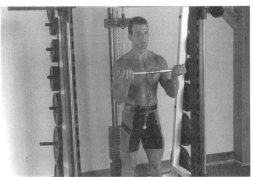

Seated Two Arm Dumbbell Curls

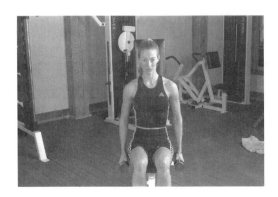
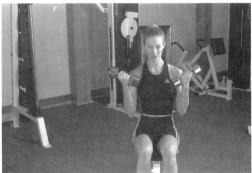

Lower Bicep Exercises

Incline Dumbbell Curls

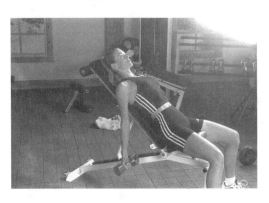
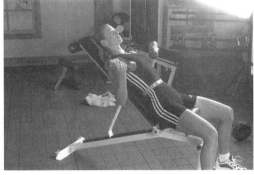

Low Pulley One Arm Curl

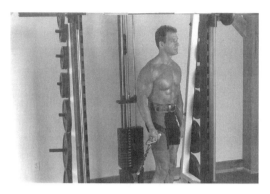
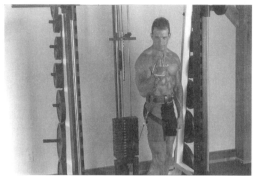

Height Of Bicep Exercises
Dumbbell Concentration Curls

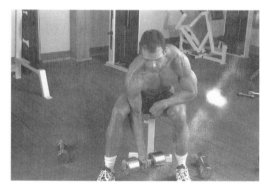
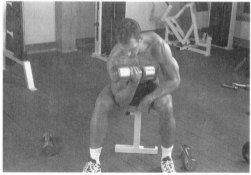

Outside Bicep Exercises
Dumbbell Hammer Curls

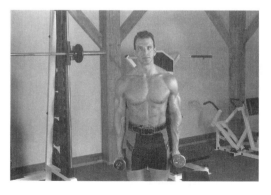
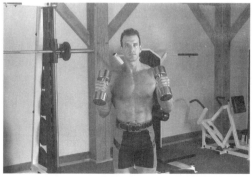

Reverse Grip Low Pulley Arm

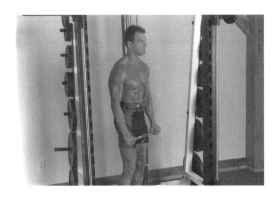
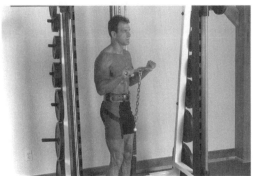

Inner Bicep Exercises
Wide Grip Barbell Curls

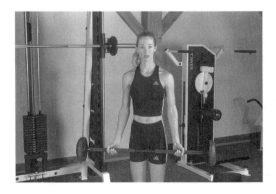
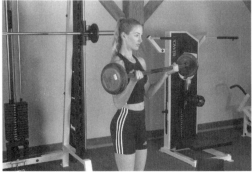

Standing Alternate Dumbbell Curls

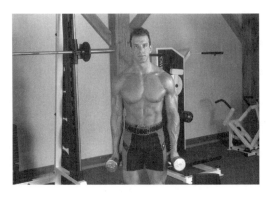
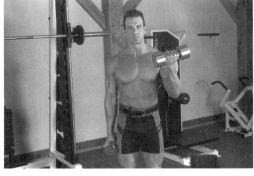

Chapter 26
More Great Exercises For The Triceps

The triceps (triceps brachii), a three-headed muscle that attaches under the deltoid and below the elbow, works in opposition to the biceps to straighten the arm and supinate the wrist. The triceps are larger than the biceps and make up about three-quarters of the upper arm.

Training The Triceps
The two ways to work the triceps muscles are pressing movements and extension movements. Even though the triceps are involved in a wide range of exercises, it is necessary, especially if you want to develop them further, to divide them into three areas: upper outer, inner, and lower part.

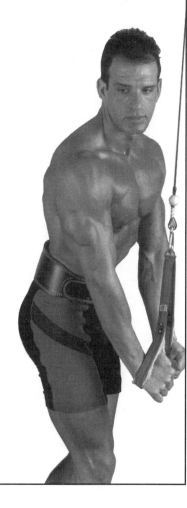

Upper Outer Tricep Exercises

Leather Strap Cable Pressdowns

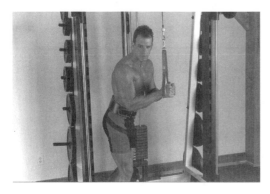
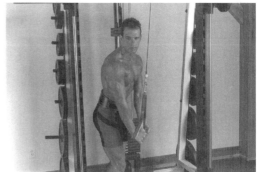

Overhead Cable Extensions V Bar

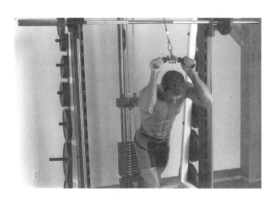
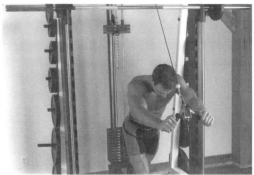

Lower Tricep Exercises

Close Grip Push-Up

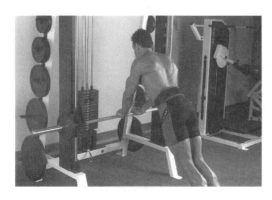
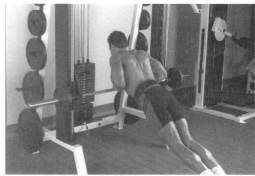

Overhead Reverse Grip Extensions

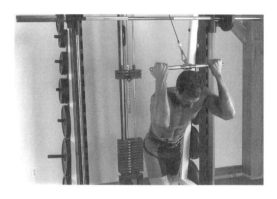
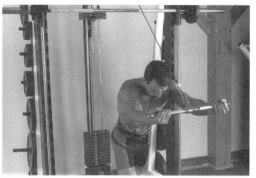

Inner Triceps

Smith Machine Overhead Press

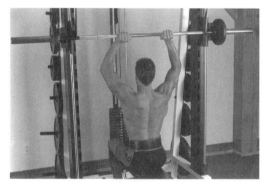
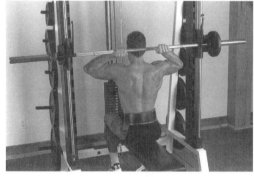

One Arm Cable Cable Extension (Palm Downward)

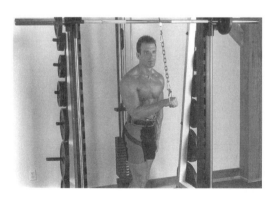
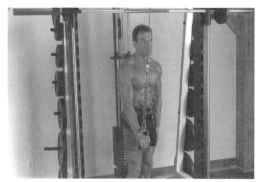

Chapter 27
More Great Exercises For The Forearms

Though often overlooked, you should consider your forearms just as important as any other body part. They are involved in nearly every upper body exercise either by helping you grip a piece of equipment or by being a part of the pushing and pulling portion of the exercise. Every time you flex the elbows or wrists, you put stress on your forearm muscles. Forearm development is important for both appearance and strength.

Anatomy Of The Forearm

The forearm is composed of a variety of muscles on the outside and inside of the lower arm that control the actions of the hand and wrist. The forearm flexor muscles curl the palm down and forward; the forearm extensor muscles curl the knuckles back and up.

Training The Forearms

Forearm training differs from other body part training because the forearms are involved in so many other body part exercises. However, I recommend that you not do as many sets of forearm exercises as you do for your legs, back, and other body parts.

The most popular way to train the forearms is by performing wrist curls. Strict technique is necessary to isolate the forearms completely in order make sure your biceps are not doing the work. You can accomplish this isolation by placing your forearms firmly on a bench with your elbows close together and locked in between your knees. If you try to do other upper body exercises when your wrists and forearms are fatigued, you will severely limit your ability to train with intensity, so always do your forearm exercises at the end of your arm training session.

Upper Forearm Exercises

Reverse Dumbbell Wrist Curl

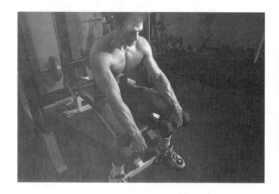 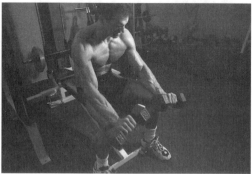

Inner Forearm Exercises

Dumbbell Wrist Curls

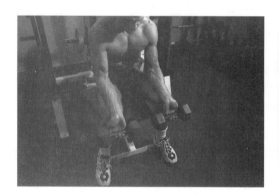 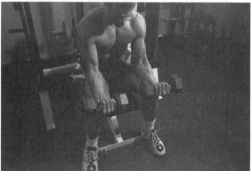

Chapter 28
More Great Exercises For The Calves

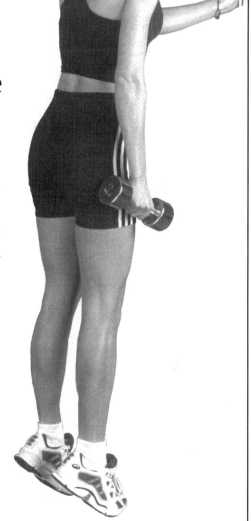

The primary muscles of the calf are the soleus, gastrocnemius, and the tibialis anterior. The soleus is the larger and deeper of the calf muscles and originates from both the fibula and the tibia. Its basic function is to flex the foot. The gastrocnemius has two heads, one originating from the lateral aspect and the other from the medial of the lower femur. Both heads join to overlay the soleus and join with and insert into the Achilles tendon which inserts into the heel bone. The basic function of the gastrocnemius is to flex the foot. The tibialis anterior runs up the front of the lower leg alongside the shinbone. Its basic function is also to flex the foot.

Training The Calves

For many the calves are one of the most difficult muscle groups to develop. They get tremendous use, when you walk or run, turn, twist, and raise up. To perform any of these movements, the calf muscles must bear all of the body's weight.

The primary exercise for the calves is the standing calf raise. This exercise works both the gastrocnemius and the soleus. The calves are tough and accustomed to much work, so the best way to get a response from them is to shock them by using a variety of exercises and training techniques.

The best way to train the calves is to divide the muscle group into three areas--lower, upper inner and upper outer—and do specific exercises that directly stress each area.

Lower Calf Exercises

Seated Calf Raise Machine

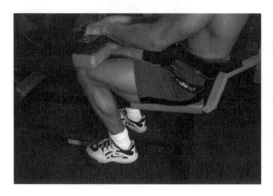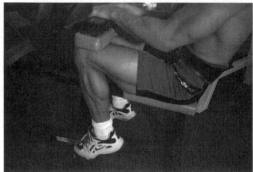

Upper Inside Of Calf Exercises

Smith Machine Standing Calf Raises—toes pointed out

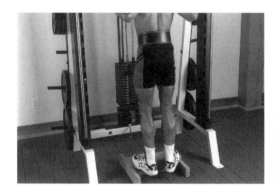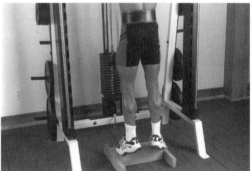

Upper Outside Of Calf Exercises

Smith Machine Standing Calf Raises—toes pointed in

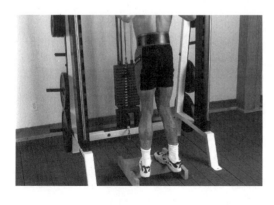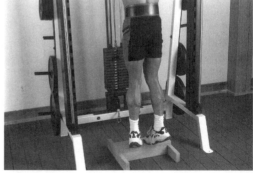

Chapter 29
More Great Exercises For The Quadriceps

The lower body is made up of more than 200 muscles. The majority of these muscles are located in the thighs, hips, and buttocks. The thigh muscles are among the largest in the human body. The main thigh muscles are the quadriceps and the hamstrings.

The quads consist of four moderately large muscles that contract to straighten the leg from a fully or partially bent position. The quadriceps are composed of four muscles at the front of the thigh—rectus femoris, bastus intermedius, vastus medialis, and vastus lateralis.

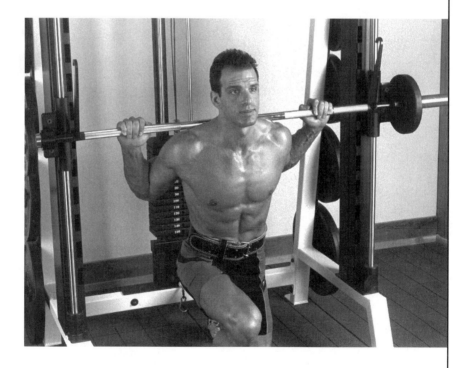

One Leg Vertical Leg Press (perform only with a spotter)

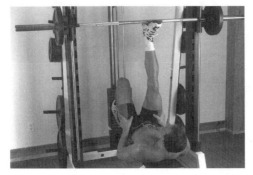 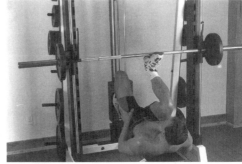

Vertical Leg Press (perform only with a spotter)

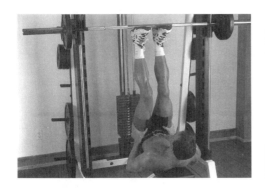 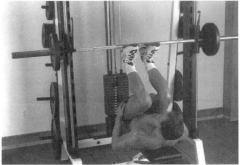

Chapter 30
More Great Exercises For Hips And Thighs

I group the glutes and upper, inner, and outer thigh together when working this area of the body. For many women this is a real trouble spot. Most women tend to lose shape, firmness, and store excess body fat in this area. These are some great exercises that target this area. Each of the exercises pictured should be repeated on the opposite side in order to work both legs.

Glute Exercises:

Multi-hip Machine (glute/hamstring)

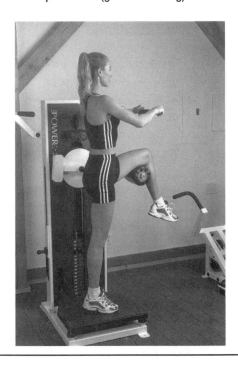
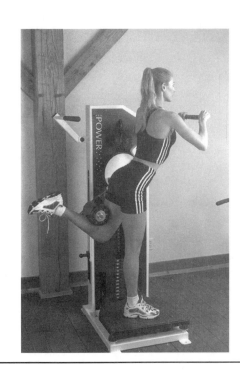

Upper Inner Thigh Exercises

Multi-hip Machine (inner thigh)

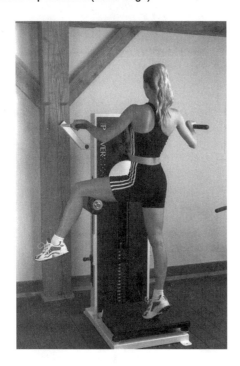 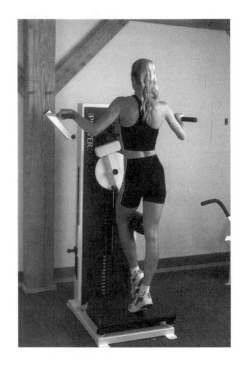

Upper/Outer Thigh Exercises

Multi-hip Machine (outer thigh)

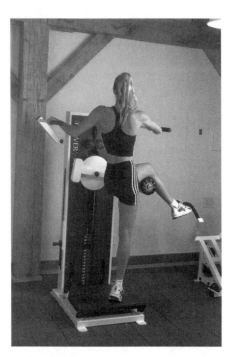 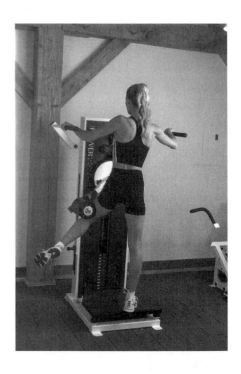

Chapter 31
More Great Exercises For The Abdomen

If your abdomen is in terrific shape, the rest of your body will be in terrific shape too. The abdomen, the visual center of the body, is composed of the rectus abdominis, the external obliques, and the intercostals.

The rectus abdominis is a long muscle extending along the length of the abdomen. This muscle originates in the area of the pubis and inserts into the cartilage of the fifth, sixth, and seventh ribs. The basic function of the rectus abdominis is to support the spinal column and draw the sternum toward the pelvis.

The external obliques (obliquus externus abdominis) are the muscles at each side of the torso (commonly referred to as the handles). They are attached to the lower eight ribs and insert at the sides of the pelvis. The basic function of the external obliques is to flex and rotate the spinal column.

The intercostals are two thin planes of muscular and tendon fibers occupying the spaces between the ribs. The intercostals lift the ribs and draw them together.

Training The Muscles Of The Abdomen

In order to achieve good abdominal development, consider the abdomen as four separate areas: the upper and lower abs, and the obliques and intercostals. By working on the abdominals in this way, you can train each area as though it was an individual body part, thus insuring great development of all areas.

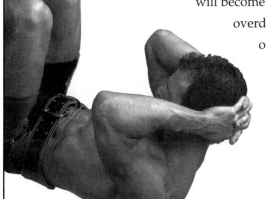

How you train your abs depends mostly on your body type. If you train the abdominal muscles with heavy weight, the muscles will become bigger and thicker. Many people actually overdevelop their abs causing them to bulge out like an inner tube around the midsection. People with small, narrow waists can enjoy success by adding weight; however, people with medium to large waists are better off not adding weight.

For the best development pick exercises that work each of the four areas—upper, lower, obliques, and intercoastals.

Upper Ab Exercises

Crunches—alternate knee touch

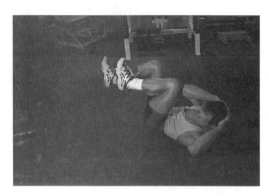 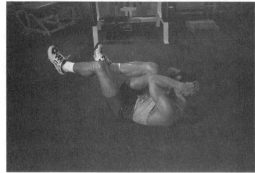

Pulley Crunches

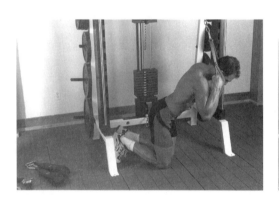 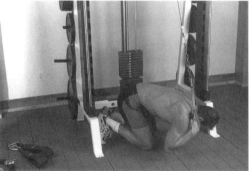

Lower Ab Exercises

Knee-ups—sitting on the floor

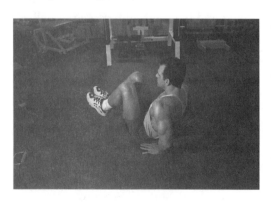 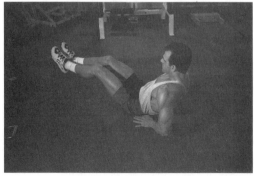

Oblique Exercises

Broom Stick Twists—seated

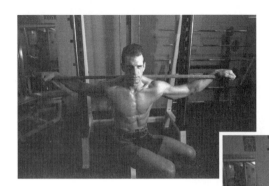

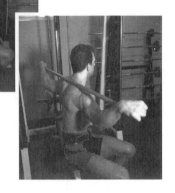

Intercostal Exercises

Hanging Leg Raises To The Side

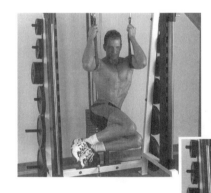

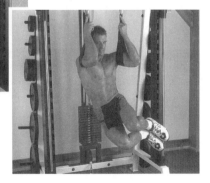

Part Three

Training For Your Favorite Sport

Everyone agrees that a well-conditioned athlete is a better performer. Getting yourself into great shape is the best way to improve sports performance and prevent injuries, burnout, and fatigue. This part of the book is dedicated to training for your favorite sport. This section is comprised of specific training programs for the most popular adult sports: running, golf, tennis, swimming, skiing, and cycling. Each of these chapters contains my favorite training routines with the recommended sports-specific exercises.

Chapter 32
Training For Running

A client that I worked with a couple years ago was a member of a running club that trained for the Indianapolis 500 Festival Mini Marathon. The members of this club ran together every day in preparation for the marathon. This year, I asked my client to continue our program but to run only four days a week. Two months before the marathon we changed his program to training his whole body with weights three times a week.

Each week, he trained twice with me and once on his own. He jogged three miles after each weight training session and four miles on one additional day per week. On this schedule, he was running twelve miles a week; whereas, most of the people in the running club were running 8, 10, or as much as 12 miles a day! The day of the mini-marathon, he shaved 35 minutes off his all-time best running record, beating everyone in the club. Training properly with weights will definitely improve your running.

Running is an activity that is aerobically demanding. Running four or five miles or more a day is great exercise. Yet, while running really gets the cardiovascular system into good shape, it does little for the muscles of the body.

The demands of intensive running add up, and in time many runners experience fatigue, weight loss, weakness, injuries, aches, and pains. Participating in a good training program which incorporates weights is a great way to ward off the negative effects of running miles and miles every day.

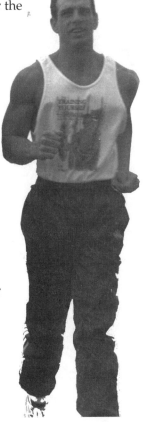

Few runners lack aerobic conditioning or are concerned with losing weight. The big concern for most runners is increasing and maintaining strength, protecting muscle mass, and averting nagging injuries.

Runners cover a lot of miles. The miles can get long and tiresome. It's important to keep this in mind when continuing your training program. It's very easy to overtrain. I like to advise runners to train twice a week with weights. This seems to be enough to maintain the conditioning levels, prevent injuries, and speed recovery if injuries do occur.

Running Training Routine
Monday, Wednesday, Friday

Monday—Upper Body
chest, shoulders, triceps, abs

Wednesday—Lower Body
quadriceps, hamstrings, calves, lower back, abs

Friday—Upper Body
back, biceps, abs

Smith Machine Bench Press

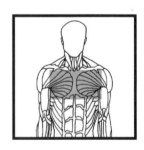

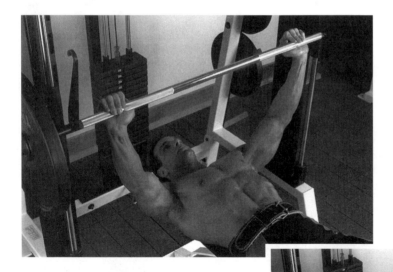

Incline Dumbbell Press

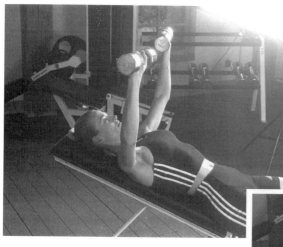
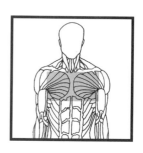
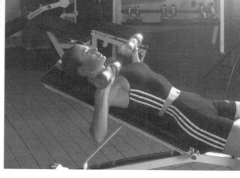

Smith Machine Shoulder Press (front of the neck)

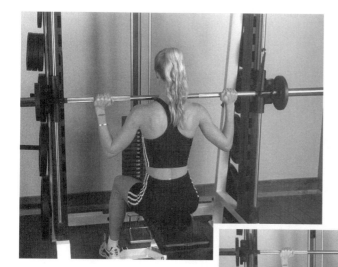
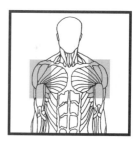

Barbell Upright Row

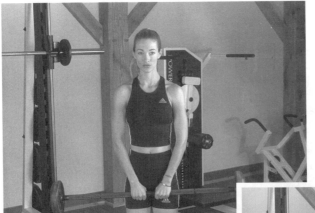
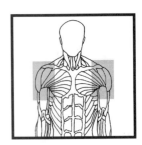
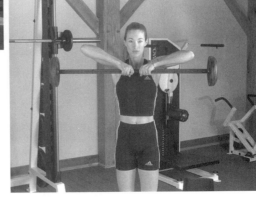

Bench Dips

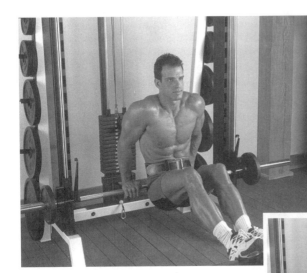
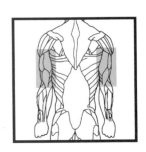

Broomstick Twists

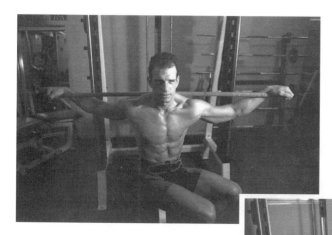
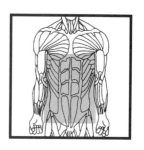

Partial Incline Sit-up

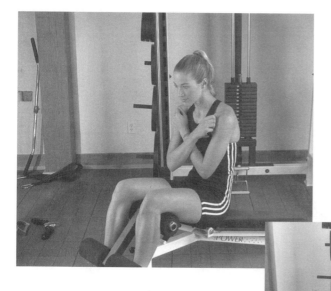
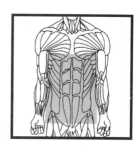

Incline Bench Knee-ups

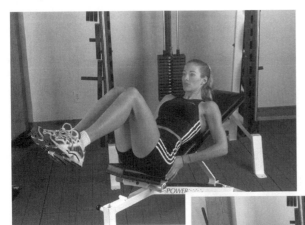
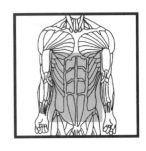

Leg Press

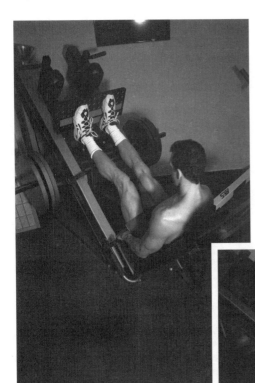
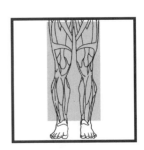

Smith Machine Squat

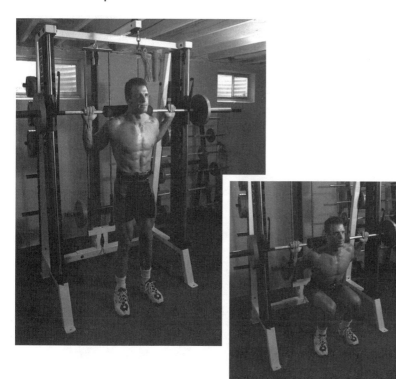

Leg Extension

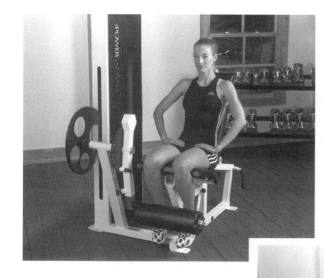

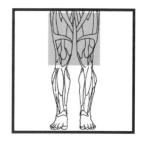

Lying Leg Curl

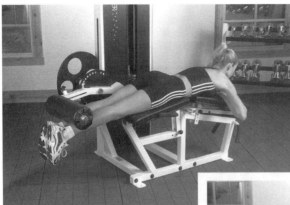
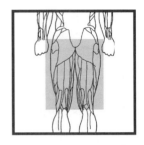
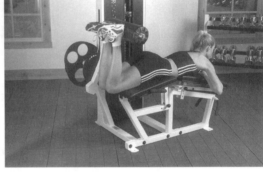

Standing Dumbbell Calf Raise

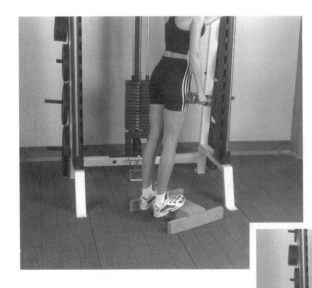
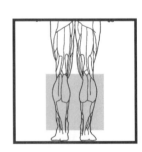

Seated Calf Machine

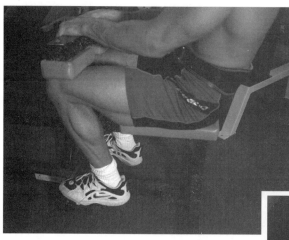
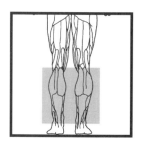
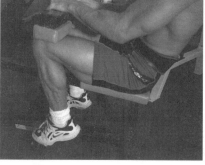

Reverse Crunch

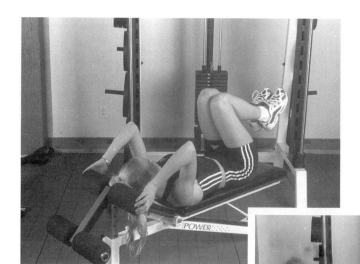
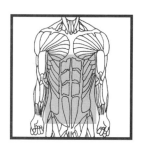

Knee-ups Incline Bench

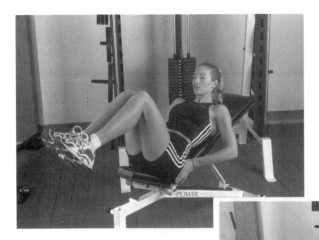
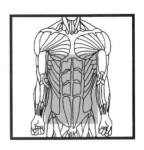

Hyperextension

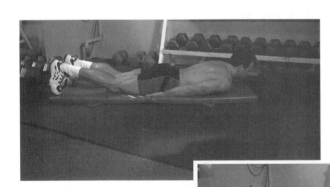
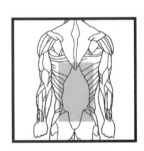

Lat Pulldown Wide Grip (behind the neck)

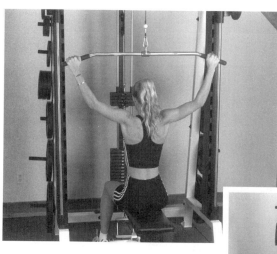
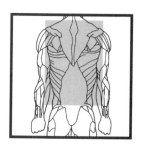
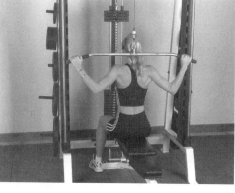

Low Pulley Cable Row

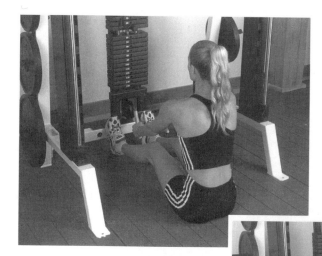
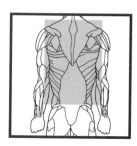

One Arm Dumbbell Row

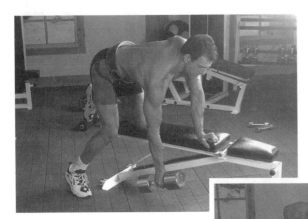
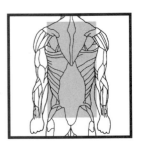
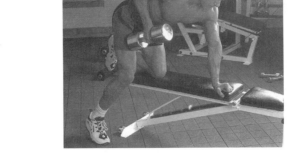

Two Arm Dumbbell Curl

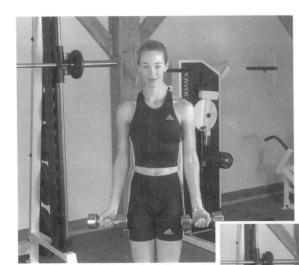
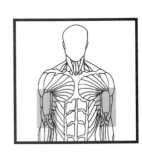

Low Pulley Arm Curl

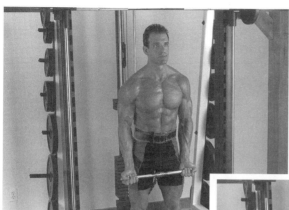
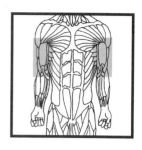
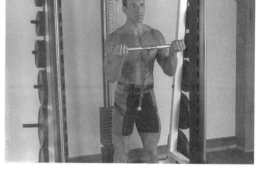

Sets and Reps
Monday/Wednesday/Friday
3 sets of each exercise
1st set 10 reps
2nd set 8 reps
3rd set 6 reps

Poundages
All Upper Body Exercises
Increase weight 5-10 pounds per set

Lower Body Exercises
Increase weight 10-20 pounds per set

Leg Extension And Leg Curl
Increase weight 5-10 pounds per set

Nonweight Assisted Exercises—
Abdominals, Hyperextensions
Exercise to Failure

Rest Between Sets
2 minutes

Techniques
Pyramid—Increase the weight for each set while decreasing the number of reps you perform. This is the best technique for building muscle mass, developing strength, and explosive power.

Stretching
Full body stretch after all weight training and aerobic sessions. (See Chapter Nine for key body stretches.)

Chapter 33
Training For Golf

When I worked for a specialty fitness equipment superstore, golf enthusiasts would come into the store almost on a daily basis looking for the latest miracle piece of equipment to improve their swing. Usually it was some apparatus that they saw advertised on late night TV. You've seen the products—miracle stretch rubber bands, the forearm flexomatic—all advertised to be the answer to improving your golf swing and driving the ball further down the green.

The mechanics of a golf swing require more than just the muscles in your forearms. It involves almost every major muscle group in the body, from the calves to your lower back and abdominals, and also your shoulders and neck. Many muscles are involved in the swinging of a club.

Golfers who want to improve their swing, as well as every aspect of their game will do best by getting involved in an overall body training and conditioning program. As in all sports, a stronger, in-shape, well-conditioned athlete will perform better.

Although golf is not a physically demanding sport, being in good shape will do a tremendous amount to improve your performance. It's important to keep this in mind when setting up your training program. I like to advise golfers to train twice a week with weights. This seems to be enough to condition the body, prevent injuries, keep flexible, and speed recovery if injuries do occur.

Golf Training Routine
Monday/Thursday—Whole Body
chest, back, shoulders, biceps, triceps, quadriceps, hamstrings, calves, lower back, abs

Smith Machine Bench Press

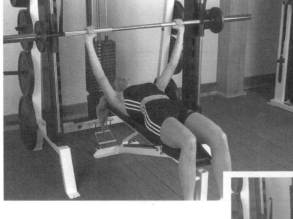
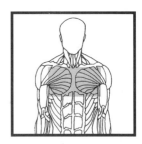
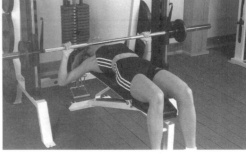

Lat Pulldown Wide Grip (behind the neck)

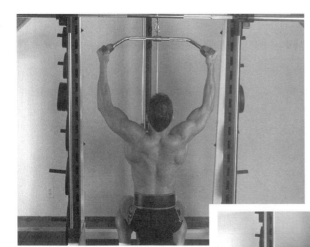
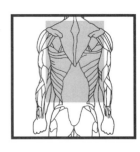

Smith Machine Shoulder Press (front of the neck)

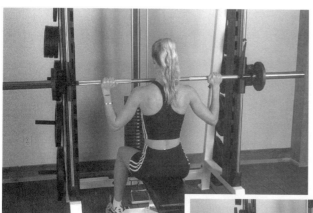
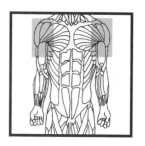
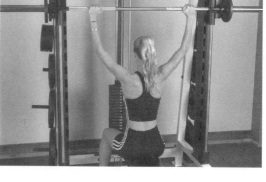

Barbell Arm Curl

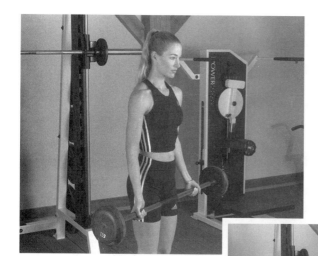
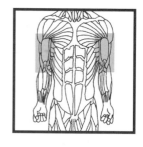

Barbell Wrist Curl

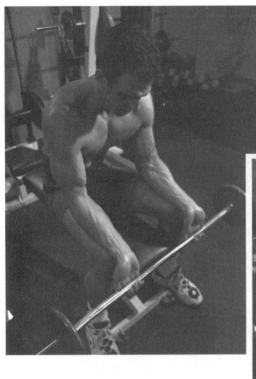
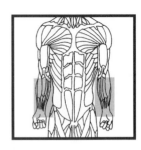
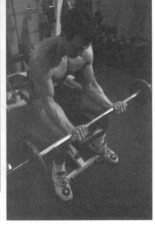

Reverse Barbell Wrist Curl

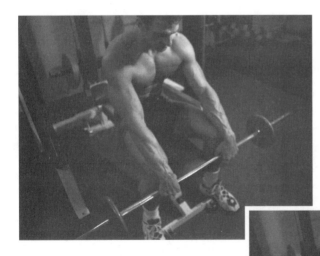
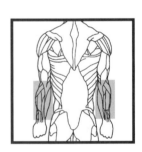

Leg Press

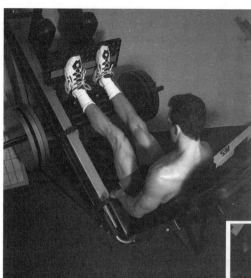
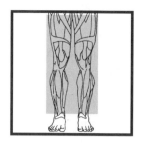
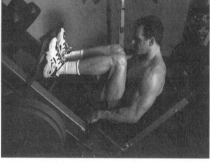

Leg Extension

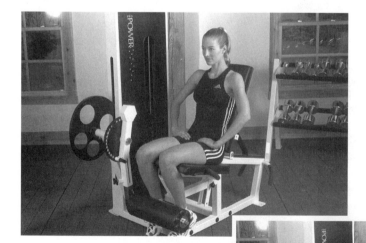
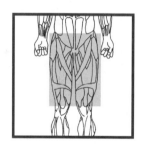

Leg Curl

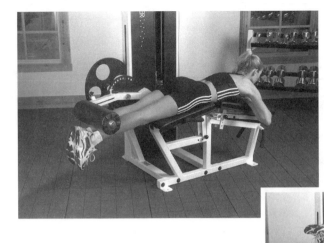
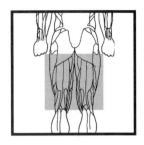

Smith Machine Standing Calf Raise

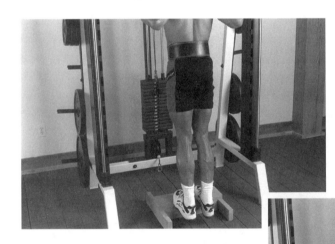
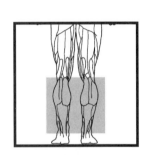

Broomstick Twists

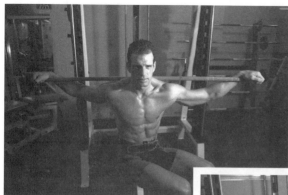
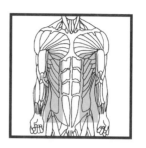
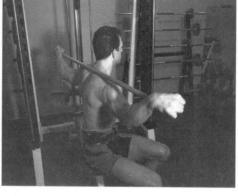

Reverse Crunch

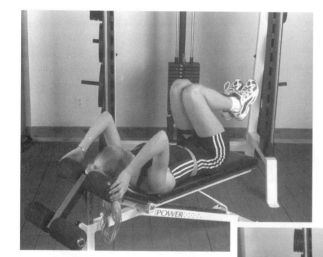
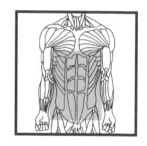

Hanging Leg Raises

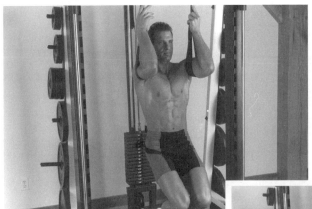
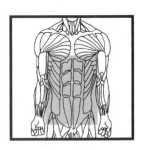
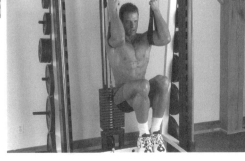

Hyperextension

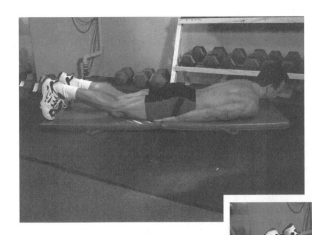
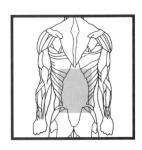

Training Sets & Reps
Monday/Thursday—2 sets of each exercise
1st set 10 reps, 2nd set 8 reps

Training Poundages
All Upper Body Exercise
Increase weight 5-10 pounds per set

Lower Body Exercise—Leg Press, Squat, Calf Raise
Increase weight 10-20 pounds per set

Leg Extension and Leg Curl
Increase weight 5-10 pounds per set

Nonweight Assisted Exercise—Abdominals, Hyperextensions
Exercise to failure

Rest Between Sets
1-2 minutes

Techniques
Pyramid—Increase the weight for each set while decreasing the number of reps you perform.

Training
Aerobic

Stretching
Full body stretch after all weight training and aerobic sessions. (See Chapter Nine for key body stretches.)

Chapter 34
Training For Tennis

Tennis is a game that requires the foot speed of a boxer, the swinging power of a baseball player, the quickness of a sprinter, and the endurance of a long-distance runner. To be a good tennis player, you have to get into great shape.

Tennis players are susceptible to shoulder, lower back, forearm, and wrist injuries. I like to incorporate special exercises to strengthen these areas.

Training with weights is a great way to improve your game. One of my clients who is 70 years old still plays tennis regularly. After training together for a couple of months, he made the comment that he was smacking the heck out of the ball, he felt quicker and lighter on his feet, did not experience as much soreness as he did before, and was able to play harder and longer and more often.

Training Routine
Monday/Thursday
Whole Body
chest, back, shoulders, biceps, triceps, forearms, quadriceps, hamstrings, calves, lower back, abs

Dumbbell Chest Press

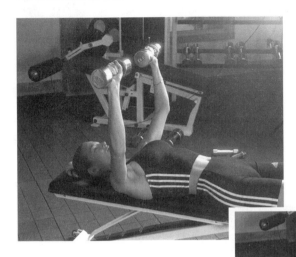
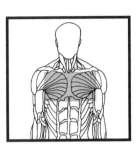

Lat Pulldown Wide Grip (behind the neck)

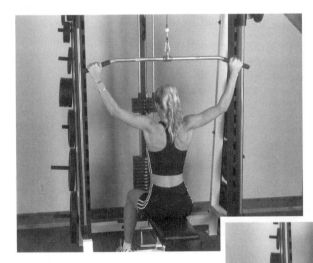
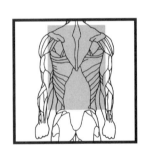

Dumbbell One Arm Press

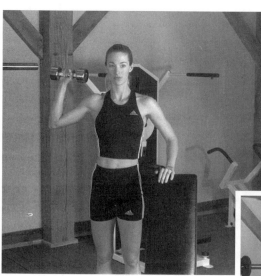
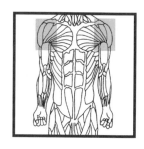
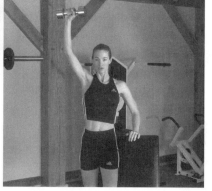

Dumbbell Lateral Raise

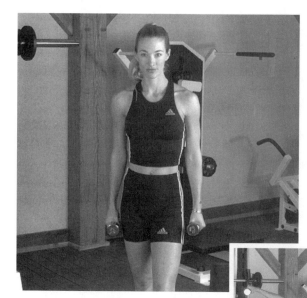
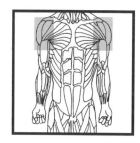

Two-Arm Dumbbell Curl

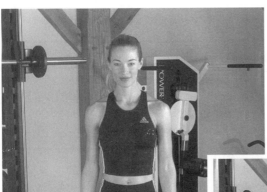
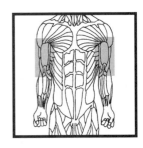
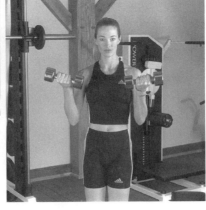

Dumbbell Wrist Curl

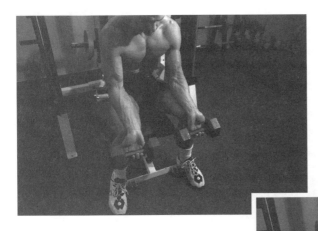
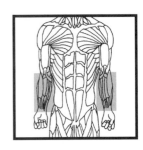

Reverse Dumbbell Wrist Curl

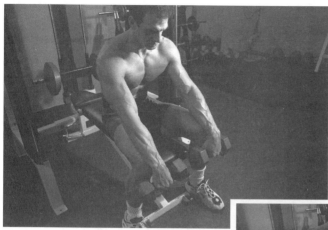
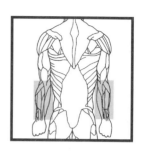
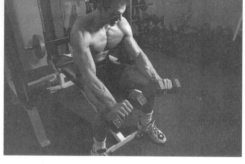

High Pulley Overhead Extension

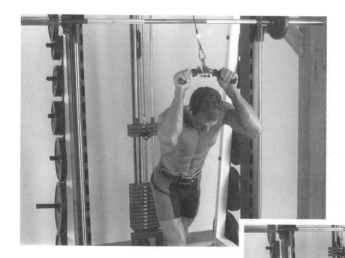
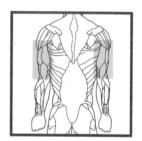

Leg Press

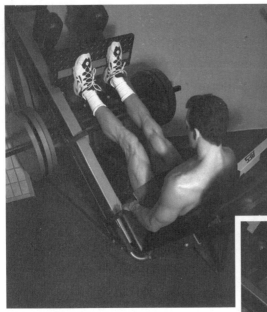
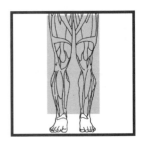
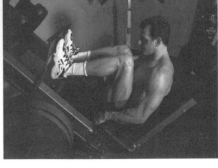

Leg Extension

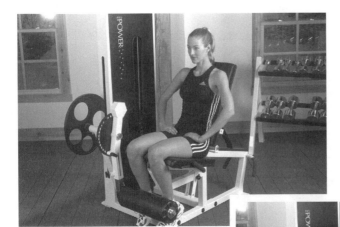
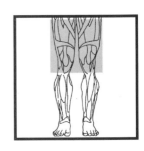

Leg Curl

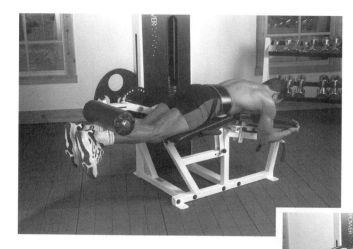
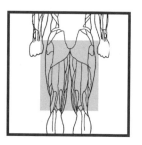

Dumbbell Calf Raise

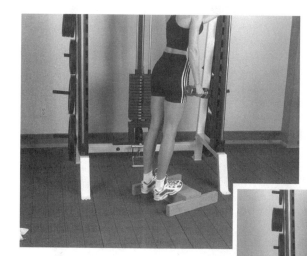
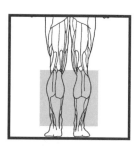

Seated Calf Raise

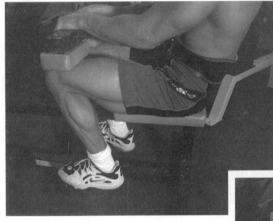
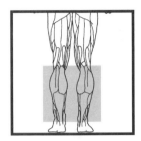
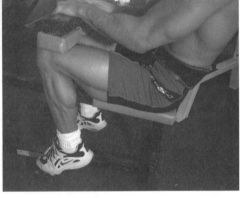

Broomstick Twists

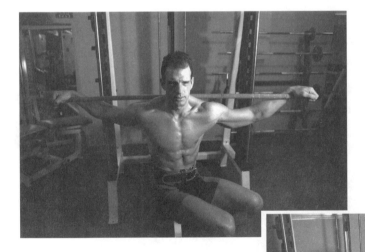
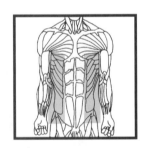

Crunch

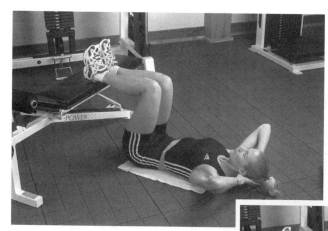
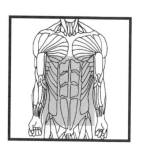

Floor Knee Ups

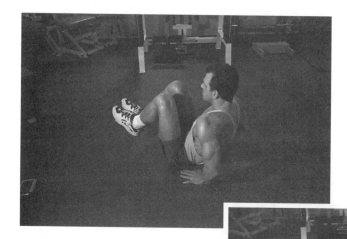
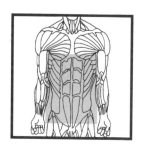

Hyperextension

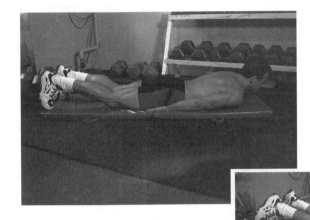
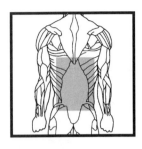

Sets And Reps
Monday/Thursday—2 sets of each exercise
1st set 10 reps, 2nd set 8 reps

Poundages
All Upper Body Exercise
Increase weight 5-10 pounds per set

Lower Body Exercise—Leg Press, Squat, Calf Raise
Increase weight 10-20 pounds per set

Leg Extension and Leg Curl
Increase weight 5-10 pounds per set

Nonweight Assisted Exercise—Neck Iso, Abdominals, Hyperextensions
Exercise to failure

Rest Between Sets
1-2 minutes

Techniques
Pyramid—Increase the weight for each set while decreasing the number of reps you perform. This is the best technique for building muscle mass, developing strength, and explosive power.

Training
Aerobic

Part Four

Getting Your Mind Into Your Training

This section is designated to help you develop the right mind set and get your head into your training. Modern psychology has taught us that the mind leads the body, that our minds produce thoughts, and thoughts govern our lives. They cause us to be who we are and act the way we do. Your body is in its present condition because, in a way, you thought it. Your thoughts actually were part of the blue prints that constructed it.

Most people make the mistake of treating exercise as a purely physical activity, figuring that all that is required to get into shape is physical exercise and a good diet. The mind, however, plays a critical role in the outcome, as in all great accomplishments. People who attempt training without building the correct mind-set don't succeed. They are the ones you see play the yo-yo game. If you want to achieve long-term success, the mental strategies covered in this section are a must. I cannot emphasize enough the importance of implementing them into your training program.

The following chapters contain information on developing a training ethic, thinking big, taking responsibility, adjusting your attitude, setting goals for your body, getting the most out of each training session, and supercharging your motivation. This section contains the tools that will empower you to turn from dreamer into achiever!

Chapter 35
Develop A Training Ethic

There are no shortcuts in training. The daily demands are firm: lifting weights, getting in aerobic exercise, and eating nutritious foods must be done consistently and conscientiously. To be successful you simply cannot get away with half-hearted, lackadaisical effort.

Training requires a commitment of time, effort, and energy. But let me quickly point out that I am not a believer in marathon training sessions.

When I was out of shape and began training, I did not have a very good training ethic. My sessions we unfocused, unorganized, and my effort was not consistent. I did not get very good results . . . and I wasted a lot of time.

Realizing that succeeding in training would not be different than succeeding in any endeavor, I decided I better develop a training ethic. The following are the steps I took to develop an iron clad training ethic. Adopt them into your program. In doing so you will find your training will become much more productive and deeply satisfying.

Step 1 Be Willing To Put Forth The Effort
Accept this now—there are no magic pills, there are no miracle thigh workers, there are no trainers you can hire that are going to magically whip you into shape. Accept right now that you are going to have to put in the effort and that a successful program will require hours and hours of training, month in and month out for the rest of your life. There are no short cuts.

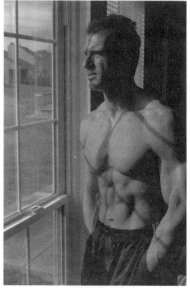

You must also accept that this is a long-term, continual commitment. There is never going to be a time when you can say, "Okay, I'm in shape. I can slack off, take it easy, skip training."

Be willing to put in the "sweat equity" up front. Many people try to squeak by only to find out that shortcuts don't pay off in the long run.

Step 2 Pay The Price

Everything has its price, even fitness. Prepare yourself in advance to pay that price.

I am always amazed at people who say they want to get into shape, and then come in with a laundry list of excuses of why they don't have the time or resources. Training requires that you make tradeoffs of time, money, and energy. It's the price of admission for an in-shape body and a healthy life.

Step 3 Become Industrious

Putting in your time is a given in achieving training success, but running up the time clock is not what I am talking about. "Putting in time" means a lot more than racking up hours in the gym.

Three-time Mr. Olympia Frank Zane says, "Intelligent training is getting the most from the least amount of effort." Be productive in your training—allocate time and then use that time in the most productive manner.

I don't like to spend more than 60-90 minutes training myself or my clients. That time, however, is productive and organized so there is not one second wasted. Organize your training program so it is as productive as you can make it.

Step 4 Eliminate Distractions

Organize your thoughts before you get into the gym. Avoid distractions and tune out your surroundings. A good way to do this is by developing a ritual to get your mind focused on your training. I have a ritual that I follow: I listen to a 10-minute motivational audio tape while I warm up on a stationary exercise bike. This helps me come down from the days events and allows me a calm period to clear distracting thoughts and get myself focused on my up-coming training session. This ritual has help me get more results, prevent injuries, and be more productive with my training.

Our minds wander from idea to idea and are easily distracted. Getting centered and focused is something you have to teach yourself to do. The better your focusing skills become, the better the results you will see in your program.

Step 5 Develop Enthusiasm

If training doesn't excite you, then more than likely you won't do it. Very few people like exercising when they first begin. It's painful, uncomfortable, and requires a lot of energy. Those who become good at it develop enthusiasm for their training. I believe this is generated by finding the value beyond just looking good or impressing your doctor.

This can also be accomplished by discovering the joy in the fundamentals. Anyone who has ever been great at something will quickly attribute their success to practicing the fundamentals. When you can shift your

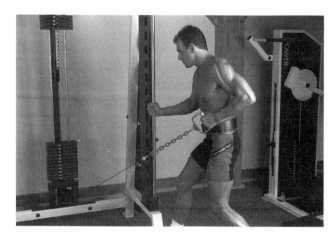

focus from the end result and learn to enjoy the process, you will become connected to the true meaning of your training and thus will become more excited about doing it.

You can also boost your excitement for training just by speaking the right language. "I get to go train" is much more positive than, "I have to work out, sigh!" The words you use influence how you view training. I always like to use the word "train" because to me "working out" implies drudgery. I am not working; I am training to improve my body, health, and life!

The greater the enthusiasm you can generate, the greater the rewards of your training program.

Step 6 Take Initiative

Initiative is a key element in any kind of performance. Simply defined, initiative is the ability to take action.

Take the initiative to control your training. Work at making necessary adjustments and changes if your program is not showing results. It always amazes me to see people staying with a losing program. If you're not getting the results you want, then take the initiative to make some changes.

When you exercise your initiative, you demonstrate the courage to make decisions and take action. This is a trait that is incredibly empowering.

Step 7 Work At Sharpening Your Skills

Anyone who has played golf understands practicing a bad swing can kill your game. When a golfer loses his swing, he loses his desire to play the game. It's the same in training. Many times people pick up bad habits and develop lousy techniques. This always leads to a lack of results and ultimately kills one's enthusiasm to train.

Getting the most out of training requires skill sharpening. Improving your training skills is a great way to get more into your training, because the better we become at something the more likely we will do it. Also, if we keep improving we are less likely to develop bad habits.

Keep your skills sharp by educating yourself. Reading books and working with a coach or trainer are great ways to stay enthusiastic and motivated. Always work at improving your skills. The better you become at something, the more confidence you have doing it, and the less awkward it feels. The better you become, the more you want to do it. In training, this equals better results.

Step 8 Put More Into Your Training Than You Expect To Get Back

A client that I worked with several years ago used to say, "I only want to put in enough effort to maintain my current level of conditioning." As you can probably guess, this person no longer trains. In fact, today this person is in very bad physical shape. The problem with the attitude of "doing just enough to get by" is that the body changes every day. We get a little older, our lives get filled with more stress, the challenges become greater. What was good enough yesterday will not be good enough tomorrow.

Legendary University of Michigan coach Bo Shembelcher used to say, "You are either getting better or getting worse." There is no middle ground. Doing just enough to get by today will set you back tomorrow.

I have found you can counter this tendency by adopting the practice of "putting in more that you expect to get back." It's an attitude of adding a little extra effort to each training session.

Make the decision right now—if you are going to exercise, then you are going to give it your all. Remember what goes around, comes around. In training you always get back exactly what you put into it!

Step 9 Develop The 3 D's (Dedication, Discipline, and Desire)

Developing dedication, discipline, and desire will not only enhance your training, but all other areas of your life:

Dedication is developed through consistency. The more consistent you are with something, the more you appreciate, savor, and relish it. Being consistent means you must also be flexible—bending but not breaking. You might alter your training program because of life's events, but you should never break it.

Discipline stems from self-control. One of the most important ways to develop self-control is through repetition. The more you do something the more it becomes "normal" and ingrained in your operating system. The key to developing discipline is habit. The more training sessions you get under your belt, the more disciplined you will become with your program. Developing discipline in training has a nice side effect—it tends to spill over into other areas of life. As I became more disciplined with my training, I found I became more disciplined in my career, commitments, and personal life. With the many different variables in training, this one element—discipline—will play the most pivotal role in your overall success.

You increase your desire for training by developing passion for it. Giving your training some excitement energizes, fuels, and powers it. It's passion to improve yourself that gets you out of bed and into the gym early in the morning.

If you embrace the principles in this chapter, you will develop a training ethic that will help you reach all your goals. You must be willing to put in the effort and pay the price, but, believe me, the benefits you reap will be better than you ever thought possible.

Chapter 36
Think Big

Can you imagine what they said when young Tom Monaghan bought a $500 mom-and-pop pizza restaurant in Ypsilanti, Michigan, and declared that he was going to turn it into the largest pizza delivery chain in the world?

Or how about when John Mellencamp quit his job working for the telephone company to form a rock band?

Today Tom Monaghan has over 5,000 Domino's Pizza stores, and John Mellencamp has sold over 40 million records.

You should have heard them laugh the day I announced I would transform my body from weighing 250 lbs. with over 25% body fat to a body that looked good enough to appear in magazines.

Today I am happy to report that this former fat boy has appeared on book covers, in TV commercials, advertisements, videos, and posters

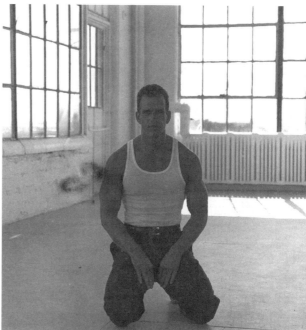

Is anything possible or are there limitations to what we can achieve?

I have found that people who achieve great accomplishments all have one similar trait—they all think big. Success and high achievement are possible for everyone, but unfortunately most people do not know how to achieve big. They remain locked out. "Thinking big" is the key that unlocks the door to all great achievement.

How about you? Don't you have some secret dream that you want to achieve? Or how about a secret fantasy of how you wished your body looked? If you want to accomplish big things with your training then you are going to have to think big.

And remember this . . . your aspirations, dreams, and big goals don't have to make sense to others. Don't seek approval from family, co-workers, or friends. Your dreams are yours!

Set some big goals for yourself in training and in life. Really go for it!

Keys for Thinking Big

-Forget about the past
In training it doesn't matter where you start but where you wind up.

-Open your mind to all possibilities
Nobody really has the answers. Nobody really knows what you can and can't achieve! There was a time when it was impossible to get to the moon!

-Do not be persuaded negatively by others
Shut the door on people who want to place limits on you. Some people don't want to invest the effort it takes to succeed, and they don't want you to, either. Often it is the people closest to us who have the most influence in holding us back.

-Don't worry about the "how." Work on cultivating a compelling "why"
When many people attempt something, they get "task worry" trying to figure out every detail in advance. This leads to unnecessary anxiety, frustration, and procrastination. To avoid this, spend your energy cultivating a compelling reason why you are doing this and everything else will fall into place.

Thinking big is nothing more than removing restraints, taking off the shackles we place on ourselves. Most of us squander our dreams in order to keep from rocking the boat, even though we know deep down inside that we have the right to be who and what we want to be, even if it isn't compatible with what others have in mind for us.

By thinking big we accept challenge. Challenge is a great motivator. It forces us to grow. Not thinking big restrains us; it immediately places limits on our potential. When we limit ourselves, we resist growing and becoming our best. In doing so we run the risk of boredom and unhappiness. Don't ever place limitations on yourself. On the contrary, think big and always fight for your dreams.

Now, set some big goals for your training and GO FOR IT!

Chapter 37
Take Responsibility

Have you ever heard someone say, "My job is getting me out of shape," or "My boss caused me to skip my workout," or "The holidays made me put on weight."

How is this possible? How can a job force you not to exercise? A job can't physically lock the door shut of the gym. How can your boss make you miss your workout? Bosses can't tie people up and hold them hostage. I have never seen a holiday physically stuff food down someone's throat.

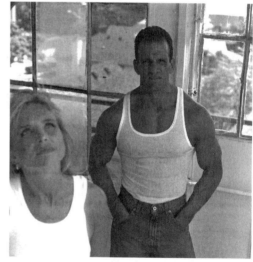

You probably hear people make statements like this every day. And you have probably done this yourself. It seems like when we are faced with responsibility, it's easier to push it off onto someone or something else. We become sort of like children who blame imaginary friends for their wrongdoings.

When we give our power away we become victims. This is a trap many people get themselves into with their health. Saying, "The doctor says I need to . . ." or "My trainer is forcing me to . . ." excuses oneself from responsibility.

Giving power away always leads to blame. When we blame others or circumstances, we give up our own sense of responsibility. Many times blame is an attempt to justify our inability to take action and produce results.

We look for things outside ourselves to blame for our lack of ability to make things happen. Blame is particularly crippling because it directs control away from the self. It puts someone else in the driver's seat of our lives.

This is very common in fitness, health, and training. People don't want to assume responsibility for their bodies. They push the responsibility off onto doctors, trainers, employers, even the school systems. How many people do you know who are letting others direct their health?

Giving your power away is a very dangerous trap.

In all honesty, no circumstance, no person, nothing can really force us to do something without our consent and involvement. But we all seem to fall into this trap from time to time. Success in training requires self-responsibility. It requires that you take control or your health, your training, your body. It requires that you claim responsibility, stand up and say, "I am in charge here. I am in control. I am responsible for who and what I am. I control my destiny."

If you are currently out of shape, being responsible means accepting that it was you who got your body in that condition.

The bottom line is you are responsible for your health, your fitness, your training, and the food that goes into your mouth. You are responsible for your body. You are responsible for your life! You are the only one who is going to get you into great shape!

Chapter 38
Adjust Your Attitude

If you want to succeed, you have to have a good attitude. There's no getting around it. No matter what you're trying to achieve, your attitude will play a huge part in whether or not you are successful.

Having a wild-eyed, super-charged positive outlook is not what I am talking about here. Yes, in order to succeed in your training you will have to have a positive mind set, but there is something much more important than being able to look at a glass of water and see that it is half full, not half empty. Most people fail with their training programs from the start because they have the wrong attitude. It's not that they aren't positive about doing their workout, or that they are not charged up to give it their all, but their mindset is missing an important element. This element is the "Attitude of Become." It will be the difference between success and failure for your training goals.

Let me explain this attitude. Once in an interview, the interviewer asked me why I have been able to succeed at changing my body when most people who attempt to change their bodies fail. I told my interviewer, "Success in training is dependent upon having the right attitude, the 'Attitude of Become.' When I decided

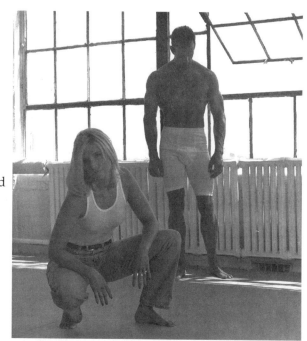

to get my 250-pound, overweight, and out-of-shape body healthy, the first thing I did was develop this attitude. By definition, 'attitude' means a way of thinking and 'become' means to develop into, change into, turn into, assume the form of. It was a totally new mindset that boiled down to this: You have to mentally create the identity of who and what you want to become. You have to mirror what you want to attract before you can gain it."

If you want a fit, healthy body in reality, you have to become a fit, healthy body in your thoughts and habits. When I first set my goal to get into great shape, I asked myself, "How does a person in super shape think, function, and act? What are their habits? What do they eat, how do they train, how do they treat themselves?"

The day I set the goal of getting my body into great shape, my thoughts immediately became those of a person already in great shape. My mind was ahead of my body, showing my body the way. Every action from that moment on was created from the mindset of a fit, healthy person. There was no more laziness, overeating, drinking, skipping exercise sessions, hanging out with friends who were destroying their health, or being around people who were not a positive influence on me.

Most people treat health and fitness as something you work to reach or acheive. What I have discovered, however, is that it is not something you can pursue—it's something you must become. James Allen said, "People do not attract that which they want, but that which they are."

As you start a new training program or revamp an existing one, plant this very important seed in your mind—the "Attitude of Become." Mentally create the identity of who and what you want to become and begin mirroring what you want to attract. As Gandhi said, "You must become the change you seek."

Chapter 39
Goal Setting

Most of my new clients seem surprised when I ask them about their fitness goals. They think it's a strange idea to set goals for their bodies. But why not? You set financial goals, career goals, personal goals. You set goals every day that you don't even think about. You set a goal to be up by 6:00 in order to make it to work by 8:00. So why not fitness goals? Your body, like a business, needs goals to grow and prosper.

Let me say up front that you don't have to be afraid of setting your goals in terms of appearance. We often think exercising for health is OK, but exercising to look better is vain. But deep down, what goal motivates you more—lowering your cholesterol count or having a body that turns heads? If your goals are more health oriented, that's fine, but don't be ashamed of setting goals that involve how you look.

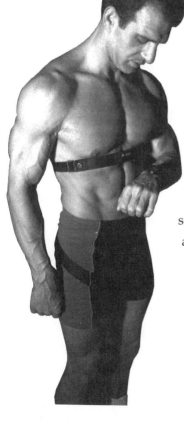

What Has Worked For Me

This is how I set goals for myself and how I help clients set their goals. I follow a three-layer format of ultimate goals, long-term goals, and short-term goals.

First, I set ultimate goals. This is the big picture. Where do you want to be in 40 years? I tend to set my ultimate goals by decades. I have in my mind what shape I want to be in when I'm 40, 50, 60, 70 and so on. I have studied people in great shape at those different ages, and they help create the shape I want to be in at those ages.

Most people skip ultimate goals. They don't think in specific terms about what kind of shape they want to be in 10 years from now. This is important because your long-term and short-term goals are pulled from your ultimate goals. In order to reach an ultimate goal 10 years from now, I set long-term goals broken down into years. Each year I set in my mind what I want to accomplish. Then from the long-term goals, I set up the short-term goals that I will need to reach in order to hit the long term goals. Short-term goals are what I want to accomplish each training season.

Reaching Goals One Step At A Time

To recap, first I set ultimate goals of 10 years. Then I list the things I will need to accomplish in order to reach those ultimate goals. Those become long-term goals that I set each year. Again, I list the things I will need to accomplish to reach those long-term goals. Those become short-term goals that I set for each training season. This can be thought of in terms of building a house. The house its self is the ultimate goal. A house is made of many different rooms. Each room is a long-term goal. Each room is built out of separate walls. Each wall is a short-term goal. Each time you accomplish a short-term goal, you have put up a wall. Each time you finish a room, you are that much closer to your ultimate goal of a house. Each smaller goal still works toward the larger, ultimate goal.

Emulating a person is a fine goal. My ultimate goal is to look like what Frank Zane looked like when he was 40. A long-term goal to reach that would be to train four times a week and not miss a workout all year. Other long-term goals are to keep my diet clean and to reduce unnecessary stresses in my life. Now the short-term goals get more specific. They are involve the day-to-day choices I make, such as phasing out soft-drinks in the next three months or targeting my abs this season.

Setting goals for your body is a very personal thing, but it is very important. The information shared here will be built on in Chapter 41, "Supercharging your Motivation."

My goals are set in decades, years, and seasons. That might not be the cycle that you choose to work in. That's OK, the structure is still the same. Ultimate goals, long-term goals, and short-term goals will work for other time frames. The point is to make you think in specific terms about where you want to be, how you will get there, and what daily choices will take you there. This goes beyond just shaping up for swimsuit season. This method of goal-setting will keeping evolving throughout your entire life!

Chapter 40
Getting The Most Out Of Each Training Session

People always comment that I must spend hours every day training to keep myself in such great shape. I don't. Successful training is not about the quantity of training but the quality of training. With two businesses and three kids, I simply don't have extra hours to spend exercising. Instead I make the time I do have to exercise count.

Mental Training Skills

Developing and applying the following six skills to your training will guarantee elevating it to a higher level. Learning and applying these skills will help you get the most out of your training.

Skill 1. Ability to Make a Commitment
Skill 2. Ability to Plan
Skill 3. Ability to Focus
Skill 4. Ability to Absorb
Skill 5. Ability to Reflect
Skill 6. Ability to Redirect

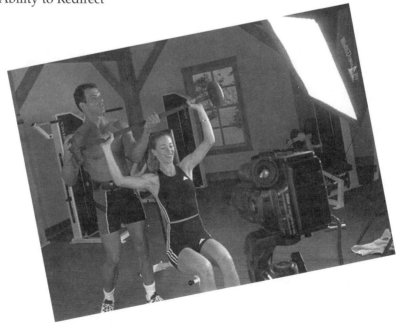

Let me explain to you how this works.

The first thing I had to do to get my body in to great shape was to **commit** 100% to that goal. That meant dedicating time, energy, effort, and a financial investment. Without a 100% commitment, it's easy to quit when the going gets tough and obstacles threaten your success. Committing also means getting away from people and activities that don't support your best interests. It means saying goodbye to some old friends and making room for new ones that will share and support the success of your goals. It means re-establishing your priorities and eliminating activities from your schedule that may interfere with your progress.

Without a **plan**, you can't accomplish anything. It's like getting behind the wheel of a car without a destination in mind. You end up nowhere. Developing a plan is really the same thing as having a guide. It will show you what needs to be done and how to do it. I had to develop a plan to follow to get into great shape. That plan became my daily guide or training program.

It's impossible to be in two places at the same time. A wandering mind never accomplishes anything. Developing the skill to be able to **focus** on what you are doing when you are doing it is the way you get maximum performance. In other words when you're training, your mind should be in the same room with you.

When I was first starting to exercise to get back into shape, my mind would often wander and I would lose focus on what I was doing. The end result was that my training sessions were not productive. But with effort, I was able to develop my concentration skills to the point where they are as effective as harnessing the power of sunlight through a magnifying glass to burn a leaf.

Absorbing or connecting to your performance is the way you get into what is called the "zone." This is that place that peak performers slip into when they are totally connected to what they are doing. It's when effort becomes effortless, and performance is perfect. It's when all the balls you throw magically go through the hoop.

Developing the skill to **reflect** each training session, both the good and the bad, is how you learn what needs to be adjusted and improved. Reflecting is sort of like watching and reviewing the tapes of your performance.

Developing the skill of mentally video taping your performances will give you all the information you will need to make improvements as long as you have the ability to **redirect**. Redirecting is simply the skill of taking lessons learned in previous experiences and applying them to the next performance. Mentally reflecting over my training sessions always gave me valuable feedback, but the feedback was of no value until it was put to use. Taking the valuable feedback gained from reflecting and redirecting will make you more successful.

Success in training is related to performance. Apply these keys to each training session and you will set the most out of your efforts.

Chapter 41
Supercharging Your Motivation

What is the secret of motivation? Why is it that a few people can start a training program and change their lifestyle for good, while most people quit exercising within a few months or even weeks? What do I do differently that has kept me training all these years? What have I been able to share with clients that has kept them motivated and successful in their programs?

What is the secret?

Motivation is not something some are born with and some aren't. It is something that can be developed and utilized to make you successful in all areas of your life, not just in training.

How well a client will do in their training can be determined strictly by what I am going to talk about in this chapter—their level of motivation.

Success in training is not dependent on genetics, experience or current level of conditioning. What determines one's potential for training success is their level of drive to improve. Their level of commitment and their enthusiasm. They feel the need to achieve, to become something more.

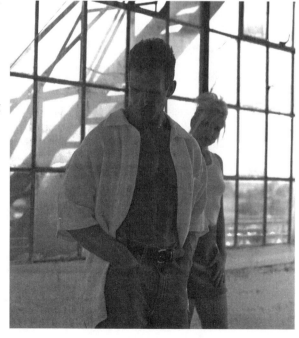

Motivation Is Energy

A simple definition of motivation is that motivation is energy. How can one be motivated to get to the gym, lift those weights, run those miles without any energy? Energy is the essence of training success.

The Motivation Cycle of Training

Involving yourself in a training program sets up a natural circle of activities that work in harmony to continually fuel your motivation. In training you start with the psychological need to improve, which leads to diet and exercise, which increases energy, which enhances performance, which improves commitment and drive, which starts the cycle over again. It is a circle of activity that feeds upon itself. Take out one element, and you break the cycle and stop the process. When someone says they lost their motivation, it's because this cycle or chain was broken.

Is There Any Passion In Your Training?

One of the first things to look at with your training program is whether there is any passion behind it. If not, then a red flag should go up—something is wrong or lacking. If the passion to improve yourself isn't there, then you need to take a hard look at your life. A training program that lacks purpose and passion will never be able to ignite spirit and become alive. It's this very important spirit that will turn passion into motion.

Think of it this way: Training motivation is really a passion for life, an emotional drive to improve the quality of your well being. This passion for living, this rush of doing something of quality, is what gets you fired up to lift those weights and run those miles. But you can't get this rush unless you develop a drive to improve yourself. This is where most people are failing with their programs; they have no passion or purpose behind their training.

Motivation Involves Risk

Did you know that motivation involves risk and that many training programs fail because they lack an element of risk? Now the risk I am talking about is not of physical nature. The risk I am talking about is the risk to improve, to change, to become.

Training involves change and change always involves risk. Staying where you are, being what you have always been involves no risk. Most people won't take the risk of not making it, of disappointing themselves. Making changes means stepping out, moving to the front of the class, risking the comfort of the backyard. But change can't happen without risk, and motivation can't be fueled when you're content with the status quo.

In training you have to go beyond your current boundaries. You have to risk where YOU are with where YOU are going to be in the future. You must strive to better yourself by pushing beyond your current limits. If you stop, you stagnate.

Motivation is fueled by energy and risk. Energy and risk are the cornerstones of performance. That's how it happens.

The Wrong Way To Motivate Yourself

Many people start training because of fear—fear of health problems, lost love, whatever. But let me warn you—motivation out of fear is not a good idea. Why? Because fear causes you to focus on the future tense. Although it might work initially, over time fear will undermine your commitment because fear takes the fun out of training. Fear undermines the sense of joy in doing something and this cripples motivation.

Fear motivation is future-based, and you cannot live in the present when you're focused on the future. Our best and most enjoyable experiences are always when we are tuned into the present moment, enjoying the process. Fear takes you out of the moment and ties you only to the future outcome.

When training, you need to focus on enjoying the process and getting connected to the training itself. Get into the "doing" instead of postponing your feelings into some future time. Don't think, "When I lose those 10 pounds, I will finally be happy." It doesn't happen that way. You will lose 10 pounds and still find yourself unhappy.

What you really need to do is find a sense of fulfillment and accomplishment in your training. Do the very best that you can and whatever happens, happens. If you enjoy the process, that's what matters. What is really important is that you set the stage for getting into the process of training and not be strictly bound to the outcome.

Conclusion

When you really analyze motivation, it comes down to a passion to improve yourself. It is important that you come to this different understanding of what motivation is. Most of us have been taught to believe that motivation is something we can gain from outside of ourselves—a product or a pill. Or we think we aren't motivated because we don't have "it" or we haven't set the right goals or worked with the right trainer or joined the right club or picked the right goal.

But motivation has to come from a much deeper place. It has to come from deeply rooted psychological needs way down deep inside—the place that defines who you are and what you want to be.

TRAINING YOURSELF

About the Author

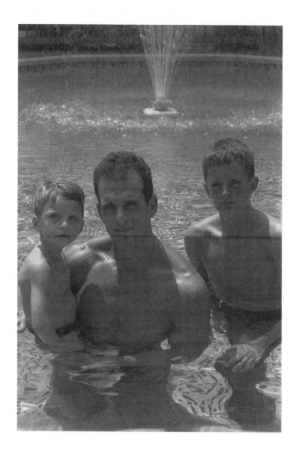

Kris Gebhardt is the author of a collection of books on physical training, personal fitness, peak performance, and personal development. His mental and physical approach to excellence revolves around training for "self development"—developing the whole person in body and mind. His books uniquely blend all the important aspects of personal growth. This makes his books a must-read not only for those who wish to changes their bodies and get into the best shape of their lives, but also for those who wish to become peak performers and experience the best life has to offer.

Other Books by Kris Gebhardt

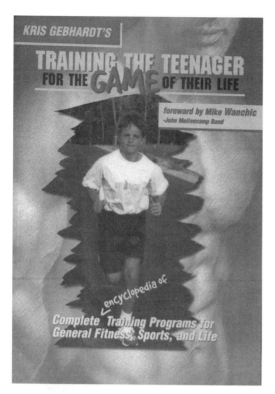

Training the Teenager
480 pages • 7 x 10 • paper
b/w photos
1-891947-00-1 • $18.95

Teaches teens how to get fit and train for their favorite sport. Includes sections on general fitness, including aerobic training, weight training, nutrition, figure firming for girls, safe weight loss; training for a variety of school team and individual sports; and total mind training, including visualization, self-talk, goal setting, positive attitude and more.

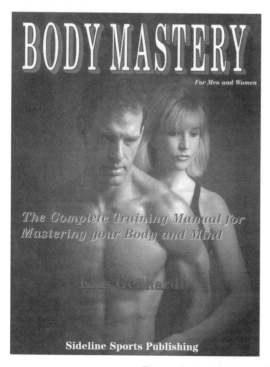

Body Mastery
228 pages • 8½ x 11 • paper
b/w photos
1-890073-00-8 • $17.95

Best of the Backlist '97, '98, & '99

Learn how thoughts, feelings and actions create the body. This book explains the concept of "Intelligent Training," the process of enacting physical change through development of the whole person. It's a must-read for anyone who wants to get into great shape and experience the best life has to offer.

For ordering information visit our Web site:
www.gcipress.com
or 1-800-643-2412

The Professional Series P.T.S. is the most innovative training system available.

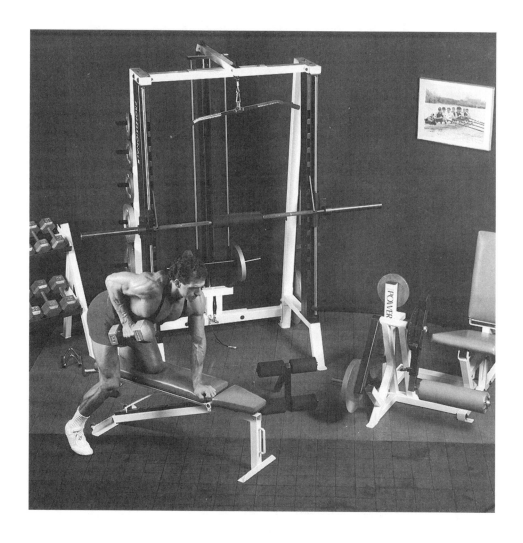

For information please
call 1-800-643-2412
or visit
www.gcipress.com